T0102133

"*Brilliant, visionary, accessible. Reveals how VNS can promote immunity, revolutionize medicine, and change the world!*"

—Marie-Ève Tremblay, PhD, College Member
of the Royal Society of Canada

THE
VAGUS-IMMUNE CONNECTION

Harness Your Vagus Nerve to Manage Stress, Prevent Immune Dysregulation, and Avoid Chronic Disease

JP ERRICO
(COFOUNDER OF ELECTROCORE)

Text copyright © 2024 JP Errico. Design and concept copyright © 2024 Ulysses Press and its licensors. All rights reserved. Any unauthorized duplication in whole or in part or dissemination of this edition by any means (including but not limited to photocopying, electronic devices, digital versions, and the internet) will be prosecuted to the fullest extent of the law.

Published by:
Ulysses Press
PO Box 3440
Berkeley, CA 94703
www.ulyssespress.com

ISBN: 978-1-64604-619-5
Library of Congress Control Number: 2023943928

Printed in the United States
10 9 8 7 6 5 4 3 2 1

Project editor: Renee Rutledge
Managing editor: Claire Chun
Proofreader: Sherian Brown
Front cover design: Rebecca Lown

IMPORTANT NOTE TO READERS: This book has been written and published for informational and educational purposes only. It is not intended to serve as medical advice or to be any form of medical treatment. You should always consult with your physician before altering or changing any aspect of your medical treatment. Do not stop or change any prescription medications without the guidance and advice of your physician. Any use of the information in this book is made on the reader's good judgment and is the reader's sole responsibility. This book is not intended to diagnose or treat any medical condition and is not a substitute for a physician. This book is independently authored and published and no sponsorship or endorsement of this book by, and no affiliation with, any trademarked brands or other products mentioned within is claimed or suggested. All trademarks that appear in ingredient lists and elsewhere in this book belong to their respective owners and are used here for informational purposes only. The author and publisher encourage readers to patronize the quality brands mentioned in this book.

CONTENTS

PREFACE

Ali Rezai looked at me and offhandedly said, "If cutting a nerve provides a clinical benefit, stimulating it could provide the same benefit without permanently destroying it." Twenty-five years later, the words of Rezai, the world-renowned functional neurosurgeon, still echo in my mind. In fact, that comment and its deep consequences have defined the past two decades of my career. In the pages that follow, I hope to share some of what I've learned, and in the process teach you how to be a happier, healthier, and smarter person, with a longer and more productive lifespan.

In 1995, I was recruited out of graduate school (for both engineering and law) by my uncle, Thomas Errico, also a world-renowned surgeon, to help him develop new spinal implants. He and I went on to cofound a series of successful companies. Three years into our first venture, he introduced me to Ali. In the late 1990s, although still in his thirties, he was performing deep brain stimulation procedures to treat Parkinson's disease. What I saw during these cases was awe-inspiring. His patients arrived for the surgery trembling uncontrollably. The procedure began by drilling screws into their skulls to immobilize their heads within a metal frame. Even with their skulls forced to be still, their arms and hands still shook incessantly. The patients were kept awake as tiny electrical leads, or wires, were inserted deep into their brains. For hours on end, Ali and his team would gently move the electrode into various positions, trying to find the magical spot. When Ali and the team reached it, like a defibrillator for the brain, the tiny jolts of electricity would utterly stop the shaking. In an instant, the patients who had been locked in torment were suddenly released. It was the closest thing to magic I had witnessed in medicine, and to this day, the effects of neuromodulation are often awe-inspiring with their speed, efficacy, long-term effect, and nearly total safety.

Ali was excited to meet me because he had come up with a new approach to treating palmar hyperhidrosis (excessively sweaty palms), which can be debilitating when severe, and he wanted to work with me to file patents for the idea. Palmar hyperhidrosis involves an imbalance in the autonomic nervous system (ANS) that controls the sweat glands in the hands.

The ANS is the part of your body that controls things without your conscious decision. It has two "arms": the sympathetic and parasympathetic. More specifically, the sympathetic arm drives our fight, flight, and freeze modes, also known as the "stress responses." The parasympathetic arm drives the rest, digest, relax, and restore modes. Nerves from each side often meet at structures called ganglia, nodes, or plexuses, where they work together to regulate obvious things like heart rate, digestion, pupil dilation, and kidney function. Functions like breathing, blinking, swallowing, and passing waste are also under at least partial control of the ANS. Surprising though it may seem, the ANS also exerts very strong influence over the immune system, cellular metabolism, fertility, and even the pace that we age, how smart we are, and whether or not our children are going to experience conditions ranging from childhood asthma, to middle-age weight gain, and even to dementia in old age.

In brief, Ali knew that palmar hyperhidrosis is caused when sympathetic nerves are overly active. Medications that block sympathetic activity can treat the condition, but if they don't work, neurosurgeons can be called upon to ablate, or destroy, the sympathetic nerves. Ali was rightfully concerned that destroying these nerves could disrupt organ function. His solution, in keeping with his advice, was to stimulate the nerve to gain the same effect without interrupting the rest of the sympathetic messages.

By this time, I was hooked on neuromodulation. So, in 2004, shortly after selling one of the spine companies where I had been the CEO, with nothing more than a vague sense of excitement, my business partners and I dove in. Of course, our new company needed a novel idea to pursue. With little more to go on than Ali's advice, I found myself sitting in my home office one Saturday afternoon, searching Yahoo! for "cut nerve," looking to find an example of a clinical benefit.

A first example came when I found a report from 1969, in which the researchers studied the role of the vagus nerve in the reaction to anaphylaxis in rabbits.[1] They separated the sensitized animals into two groups: 1. controls that were exposed to eggs promptly experienced anaphylactic reactions and died; and 2. test animals that had had their vagus nerves (the vagus nerve is the primary component of the parasympathetic arm of the ANS) cut before the egg exposure. These test animals had experienced a far milder reaction to the allergen and survived.

Similar studies were conducted in the US and England a few years later (in the early 1970s), but they, too, didn't follow up. It seemed like a great opportunity to restart a very interesting line of research, and, of course, I was eager to find out if nerve stimulation could produce the same lifesaving benefits.

Now, to be fair, electrical stimulation of the vagus nerve was a technology that had been developed, and implanted devices were available for the treatment of epilepsy. The original idea even dates back to the 1880s, when J. L. Corning's idea for an electrical compressor of the carotid arteries was first patented. It took a century, but Cyberonics received FDA approval in Europe for their implanted vagus nerve stimulator in 1994.

Armed with the simple hypothesis that vagus nerve stimulation (VNS) could treat anaphylaxis, our tiny company's first team went to Columbia University in early 2006. There, we conducted a series of experiments and ultimately demonstrated that VNS could prevent death from anaphylaxis. The researchers we were collaborating with were especially fascinated by the effects in the lungs. Part of the lethal cascade of anaphylaxis can be a swelling of lung tissue (called edema) and bronchoconstriction (a tightening of the smooth muscle that lines the airways). The researchers reported that these symptoms were muted or not present at all among the animals treated by our version of VNS. It was a natural segue to looking at asthma, in which both of these symptoms occur.

Confirmatory studies in animals led to full-blown clinical studies in human asthmatics who had failed self-administered bronchodilators, had come to the emergency department, and were still failing treatment with nebulized medications. These first studies had to be conducted in a hospital setting because, as of 2008, our treatment was delivered by inserting an electrode into the neck, and we weren't sure how long the therapy needed to be administered, or whether symptoms would reemerge once the therapy was turned off (if it worked at all). Needless to say, a needle jab in the neck of a patient having an asthma attack wasn't an easy procedure to encourage patients (or physicians) to consider, but over a nearly two-year period, we recruited more than two dozen patients, and the results were profoundly positive. Most interestingly, the patients reported almost immediate relief of their most challenging symptoms.

Despite the benefits, we knew we had to find a better way than a needle stick in the neck. One of my closest friends, a brilliant physicist by the name of Bruce Simon (a fellow MIT graduate, but from 1970) saved the day. He had begun playing around with a nerve conduction velocity testing machine made by a Scandinavian company called MagVenture. It was a very clunky machine that cost $80,000 and required a wheeled cart to move. It also required a significant amount of reprogramming to do what we wanted it to do, which was to stimulate the vagus nerve at 25 hertz. More importantly, however, it had the ability to deliver the signal through the skin. As much as we thought the modified device would likely treat asthma the same way the percutaneously (literally "through the skin") inserted electrode would, we needed to try it out to be sure.

As luck would have it, one of our engineering colleagues, a brilliant and hysterically funny man by the name of Jon Gardiner, was an asthmatic. Jon hated to use bronchodilator medications because they made him feel jittery. One day, late in the morning, Jon happened to be struggling with an asthma attack and jumped at the chance to try the contraption that Bruce had newly programmed to deliver our signal. In retrospect, it was probably a little crazy, but we had an anesthesiologist in the office that day, and she agreed to monitor him as he self-treated. To this day, I feel like I was present for a great moment in the history of medical science.

As Jon lifted the large paddle that contained the magnetic coils to his neck, he began to describe the sensation of having electrical currents induced by the machine, first in his ear, then his jaw, and even in his teeth. Suddenly Jon's eyes widened and he looked startled. He exclaimed, "It's gone! The attack is gone! And …," he added, as he started breathing heavily, "I can usually trigger an attack … but I can't. It's totally gone."

Armed with the knowledge that a noninvasive approach to VNS was possible, we pushed forward to find a way to optimize a delivery device. Within a year, Bruce, Jon, and several of our other colleagues had contributed to a variety of different possible devices. A few months later, a small study conducted in South Africa confirmed what Jon had first experienced.[2] By late 2011, we had landed on a safe, easy-to-use, and cost-effective way to make a noninvasive device. We called it gammaCore.

Not surprisingly, when the therapy was percutaneous, none of our colleagues, investors, family members, and friends had volunteered to try it. (In fairness, I hadn't either.) Once it was noninvasive and Jon had broken the ice, however, every one of us wanted to try it. Within a matter of a few weeks, hundreds of stimulations had been noninvasively delivered to several dozen people. The results of these random experiences were consistently encouraging, but also remarkable in the breadth of the reported benefits. For example, users with allergic congestion, or other nasal blockage, reported rapid opening of their upper airways. One volunteer even asked if the device "fixed a deviated septum," because he hadn't breathed through both nostrils at the same time in five years, that is, until he used our noninvasive VNS (nVNS) device.

Other users claimed that perimenopausal symptoms, including hot flashes and mild transient feelings of depression, were relieved. One of the most consistent and common reports, however, was that headaches present at the time of stimulation seemed simply to evaporate within minutes after the treatment.

As disappearing-headache comments began piling up, I picked up the phone and called several of the most well-respected and well-published headache specialists in the world. To my surprise and great appreciation, they answered. I shared that we had developed a vagus nerve stimulator to manage asthma attacks and were surprised to find that headaches were being successfully relieved by the therapy. The headache specialists shared that asthma and migraines often showed up in the same patients; i.e., they were common comorbidities, which means that people with one have a significantly higher than normal chance of having the other.

In fact, the specialists were not surprised at the effects we were observing, and shared that small pilot studies had already been conducted with implanted VNS devices to treat severe headache conditions. They lamented that implanted VNS devices cost tens of thousands of dollars, making it a nonviable treatment for headaches beyond pilot studies. That was my opportunity to let them know that the device we had developed was noninvasive and would be offered at far less than tens of thousands of dollars. It was handheld, and patients could self-administer the therapy on demand, as needed, as easily as taking a pill, and even more easily than self-administering an injection. They were all impressed, and many of these specialists have gone on to work with our product. They helped us immeasurably to secure the FDA clearances for the treatment and prevention of migraine, cluster headache, and a number of other severe headache disorders.

As we proceeded through the headache studies, however, I returned to the question of why a therapy that was developed for epilepsy, and had subsequently also received approvals to treat depression, was now also treating asthma and headaches in our studies. As I read more, I found other benefits attributed to VNS, in conditions ranging from fibromyalgia and rheumatoid arthritis to anxiety and Alzheimer's disease. Similarly, in our own studies, we were seeing collateral benefits, such as reducing blood pressure in hypertensive patients and normalizing glucose in those with type 2 diabetes.

As exciting as this was, it concerned me. Claims that a therapy does too much are often met with skepticism. Of course, the alternative argument is that the therapy does something extraordinarily fundamental. Willing to find either answer, we set about trying to figure out what vagus nerve stimulation really did. Having a noninvasive method made that process much easier than it would have been if we only had the use of implanted devices.

As will become obvious in the chapters that follow, we are not the only group to have studied the amazing benefits of VNS. In fact, another group that started their work just a few years before we did, in 2000, had been working less than fifty miles away from us, on Long Island, New York. Their group, headed by a neurosurgeon named Kevin Tracey, had decoded an incredibly important pathway that showed how the ANS influenced the immune system through the spleen. He termed this spleni-cally mediated pathway the *immune reflex*, and his colleagues showed how the release of acetylcholine activated a receptor (the alpha-7 nicotinic acetylcholine receptor, abbreviated α7-nAChR) on certain immune cells, especially macrophages, or specialized cells that destroy pathogens.

Many others have followed in Tracey's footsteps, discovering anti-inflammatory pathways in other organs, including the digestive tract, kidneys, and brain. In every case, the pathways boil down to the fact that stimulation of the vagus nerve moti-vates the release of acetylcholine, which acts on α7-nAChRs.

For years I have wanted to write a book describing the effects of VNS and how it can affect autoimmune disorders, metabolic dysfunction, neurodegenerative conditions, mood disorders, and pain. I consider it fortunate that I waited until now, however, because recent work has allowed me to expand the story to include the promising role of VNS in preventing neurodevelop-mental conditions, optimizing brain development, supporting healthy mitochondrial function, and even extending a person's lifespan. My deepest wish is that you will come to see the beau-tiful pattern that links all of these major areas of focus and glimpse the logic of complex life as seen from the perspective of macrophages, mitochondria, and the autonomic nervous system.

As a final note, in order to tell this story in the span of space that the publishers allotted me, I had to make some sacrifices. There are applications of VNS that go beyond the many that are discussed here. For further reading, I recommend *Activate Your*

Vagus Nerve and *Upgrade Your Vagus Nerve*, both by Dr. Navaz Habib.

CHAPTER 1

CELLULAR BIOLOGY IN A NUTSHELL

In order to understand how the autonomic nervous system (ANS), the immune system (principally macrophages), and mitochondria work together to affect pain, mood, cognitive function, metabolism, reproduction, and even longevity, we have to delve into cellular functions and even some molecular interactions. This isn't always easy for casual readers, but I am going to make you the following deal: If you do your best to remain intrepid in the face of this rigor, I will do my best to present these scientific facts in the plainest and most straightforward way possible. In addition, whenever possible, I will refresh key concepts along the way, as needed. For a few, however, it is best to simply explain them right at the beginning. Please read this chapter and, if necessary, flip back here to refresh your understanding when the concepts come up later in the text.

THE LANGUAGE OF LIFE

Estimates for the number of cell types in the human body range from a low of 150 to 200 to a high of over 400. There are more than a thousand types of cells that humans don't have, from those that produce feathers and scales, to those that produce venom or shells. Of course, the difference between a nerve cell in a human is quite distinct from a nerve cell in a nematode, or roundworm, so if we are considering the different biochemistries of cells, their number is effectively infinite.

In nearly every one of these cells, however, biochemistry and function are largely defined by inherited material made of long strings of a complex molecule, deoxyribonucleic acid, abbreviated as DNA. In fact, the most fundamental division among these cell types, which separates the tiny bacteria, known as prokaryotes, from the relatively massive cells of multicellular animals, known as eukaryotes, is how that genetic material is maintained. In the case of the prokaryotes, small loops of DNA float openly around in the inside of the cell. In eukaryotes, DNA is much more complex, and is maintained inside a nucleus as a tightly wrapped, highly organized structure.

DNA itself is composed of a pair of long polymerized sugar molecules (ribose), each connected to one of four planar organic compounds called nucleotide bases. The structure of DNA is often likened to a twisted ladder, where the polymerized sugar molecules form the twisted posts, and the nucleotide bases form the rungs by coupling together across the space between the posts. That is, the nucleotides on one post align with the nucleotides on the other. Each post spirals around the other, giving DNA the double helix appearance for which it is famous.

For all its beauty and capacity to encode secret patterns of life, the genetic code is relatively simple. There are only four nucleotide bases: adenine (A), guanine (G), cytosine (C), and thymine (T). Even more simply, in the double helix structure, adenine only couples with thymine (A-T) and guanine only couples with cytosine (G-C). Further, only one side of the DNA double helix actually contains the code (e.g., a gene), while the other side provides stability. The coded section typically consists of "three-letter words" formed by base pair triplets. Coded sections are blueprints for generating a variety of different types of useful molecules, including proteins.

The process of converting a section of DNA into a useful molecule, like a protein, begins with a copying step involving specialized protein called ribonucleic acid (RNA) polymerase that reads the encoded side of the double helix and generates a string of nucleotides mirroring the coded section. This new string is made of RNA. RNA has a similar sugar backbone (ribose) but a slight chemical difference that usually inhibits the formation of a double helix.

These strands of RNA are often modified both in the nucleus and outside (once transported there by special chaperone proteins). Following this process, one class of RNAs, referred to as messenger RNA (or mRNA), are transported to structures called ribosomes, often located within the membrane of another organelle called the endoplasmic reticulum (the ER). Ribosomes are large structures built from several proteins and special RNAs (called ribosomal RNA, or rRNA). Just as RNA polymerase "reads" DNA to produce RNA strands, ribosomes "read" the mRNA and produce strings of amino acids (also referred to as peptides). These strings of amino acids curl up on themselves in unique ways to produce proteins.

More specifically, because there are four possible bases and three letters per word, there are different possible words. Some of the words mean "start" and "stop," but the rest correspond to specific amino acids. All of life on Earth uses the same coding language, and the same words refer to the same amino acids to build proteins. There are only twenty of these amino acids, so some words have synonyms. There is one very interesting exception to this rule, which will be discussed in the context of mitochondria and cellular metabolism. Still, the ubiquitous language of life is a remarkable reminder of how similar all species, from bacteria to blue whales, are.

THE DIVISION OF CELLS

In order to better understand the origins and diversity of life, scientists often focus on differences, splitting the world into ever-smaller and ever-more homogeneous categories. The highest division of cells is into prokaryotes and eukaryotes (the more complicated ones with nuclei, lots more DNA, and organelles). The prefixes *pro-* and *eu-* mean "before" and "true," respectively, and *karyote* refers to the nucleus and the packaging of DNA therein. It turns out that eukaryotes have many organelle structures that prokaryotes don't. Prokaryotes, on the other hand, are very simple, remaining much as they existed before the evolution of organelles.

Other important differences between prokaryotic and eukaryotic cells relate to their outer membranes (and in the case of the eukaryotic cells, the membranes surrounding their organelles). The differences in the types of fatty acids used by prokaryotes versus eukaryotes allow eukaryotes to recognize potentially dangerous pathogens. More specifically, specialized proteins, exquisitely tuned to recognize and react to prokaryotic membrane fatty acids (like lipopolysaccharide, or LPS), can prompt strong inflammatory responses.

These exquisitely tuned proteins are among the class of proteins that are specially constructed to remain stable in the outer membranes of cells. Some of them change shape when they come in contact with specific molecular patterns. This shape shift allows something outside the cell to alter something inside the cell, so the cell can sense and react to something without having to incorporate it. Examples of these are often called *receptors*. In other cases, the protein residing in the membrane can open and close holes in the membrane in response to activation. These proteins are called *channels*, and they can be used to help the cell take up or release controllable quantities of molecules ranging from large proteins to tiny charged versions of atoms, called ions. Some of these ion channels can be triggered to open and close by chemical interactions, and so serve as both a receptor and a channel. In other cases, ion channels can open and close solely based on charge differences across the membrane. They are known as voltage-gated ion channels, and one of them, in particular, known as the alpha-7 nicotinic acetylcholine receptor, or α7-nAChR, plays a central role in the communications and controls of the immune system by the autonomic nervous system.

CHEMICAL AND ELECTRICAL SIGNALING

While prokaryotes can assemble into colonies and even alter their behavior in response to their position within the colony and the size of the colony, the more complicated and evolved eukaryotes are able to form multicellular organisms with far more differentiation of function. Multicellular organisms have specialized cells that have evolved to release and sense chemicals released by one another as a way of coordinating the biochemistry of the system. The molecules that similar cells use to communicate are often bundled together under one general term to distinguish them from the chemicals used by others. For example, immune cells typically communicate through a class of molecules called *cytokines*, and fat (adipose) cells release *adipokines*. Neurons typically release *neurotransmitters* to communicate with one another, and often do so by sending very rapid electrochemical signals along long tubular segments of their bodies.

More specifically, neurons have three major components: the cell body, the dendrites, and the axon. The cell body is where the nucleus (the DNA) and most of the major organelles reside (mitochondria, which will be described more fully below, are a significant exception to this general rule). The axon (there can be more than one, but one is most common) is the long tube that carries the electrical signal when the nerve fires. Dendrites are a series of finger-like structures that reach out to the axons of other neurons, connecting with them at synapses.

The firing of a neuron, also referred to as a *nerve impulse*, occurs as a result of a series of ion channels that open and close in rapid sequence. This is often initiated by neurotransmitters which cause a slow inflow of charge. A reduction in the difference between the charge outside and inside the cell can be stable until it drops to a defined level (called an excitation threshold). At this point, a series of voltage-gated ion channels open, allowing the rapid inflow of more charge. When this happens at one point, usually starting with the cell body, a cascade of ion channels opens in sequence down the axon. The rapid depolarization causes charge equilibrium to occur, and the channels close quickly. With the gradient now approaching zero, a separate set of voltage-gated ion channels open, and charge flows in the opposite direction, thus restoring the original difference in charge across the membrane. There is typically a bit of overshoot in this process, requiring the cell to rest in order to get back to its true resting state. That is called a refractory period and typically lasts several milliseconds.

The electrical activity of one nerve influences the firing of the next one through the release of neurotransmitters. The releasing cell, along with helper cells that monitor the synapse, typically take up the used neurotransmitter that is still hanging around through a process referred to as *reuptake*.

There are lots of different neurotransmitters that have been discovered and analyzed over the decades (a surprisingly large number of Nobel prizes having been handed out to folks who have done that work). Nerves often specialize in the release of one type of neurotransmitter; for example, glutamate is a particularly important neurotransmitter in that it typically causes the cell receiving it to become excited (hence it is referred to as an excitatory neurotransmitter). Glutamate-releasing neurons are often called glutaminergic. Similarly, neurons that release dopamine and GABA (gamma-aminobutryic acid) are referred to as dopaminergic and GABA-ergic neurons.

THE AUTONOMIC NERVOUS SYSTEM (ANS)

Nerves populate nearly every cubic millimeter of the body, often having long cable-like axons that span macroscopic distances (inches to feet). There are thousands of functions happening all the time, and they are under constant surveillance by the brain. These nerves make up what is known as the autonomic nervous system (ANS), and through the nerves, the brain monitors and adjusts heart rate and blood pressure, respiration and digestion, and, as we will see, the immune system and metabolism. It watches and manipulates your body without your consciously acting (or can take over for things you can voluntarily decide to do differently, like breathing and blinking, when you aren't paying attention).

As mentioned, like yin and yang, the ANS has two arms. The first is referred to as the sympathetic arm, and its largest structures are the sympathetic nerve chains that run along the front surface of the spinal bones. They form nodes at each level of the column. At each of these nodes, nerve fibers branch off and join with voluntary and involuntary fibers from the nerve roots of the spinal cord, to control all the involuntary muscles, from your heart and diaphragm to the muscles in your digestive tract. Even the smooth muscle lining of arteries and other vessels that carry lymph, urine, and all manner of other secretions are strongly influenced by sympathetic nerve fibers. The sympathetic arm is associated with fight-or-flight mode, or threat response activity.

The other side of the ANS is the parasympathetic arm, and it is composed of the vagus nerve, which descends from your brainstem along with the carotid arteries and jugular veins on either side of the neck (literally inside the sheaths that contain those critical vessels). In a similar way, nerve fibers within the vagus nerve also connect to organs and tissue, releasing its neurotransmitters to affect the function of everything from digestion to heart rate and breathing. As we will see, the vagus nerve can influence metabolism, immune function, and even blood clotting. Unlike the sympathetic arm, the vagus nerve is primarily a sensory nerve, meaning that most of it is fibers bringing information up to the brain. Activity in the vagus nerve is associated with the rest, digest, and restore mode.

The two arms of the autonomic nervous system are generally opposing forces. Not surprisingly, the neurotransmitters they release are different. Sympathetic neurons generally release norepinephrine. The parasympathetic fibers that descend into the body release acetylcholine, making them cholinergic nerves.

The ANS can be considered a third component of the immune system. Typically, however, the immune system is thought of as having two primary subsystems: an innate component and an adaptive one. The former reacts to threats and injuries with a robust inflammatory response that is, frankly, somewhat indiscriminate and can make you sick even as it is trying to defend you. The innate immune system fights chicken pox the first time you encounter it, and along the way, you feel sick. Adaptive immune cells learn from prior encounters and build very specific tools (e.g., antibodies and T-cells) that are able to rapidly destroy pathogens that are encountered a second time. It reacts so quickly and precisely that there is no getting sick from the battle.

Now, in this context, consider the role of the brain and nervous system. The network of nerves and their support cells enable us to react to situations in a way that prevents us from being injured or coming into contact with things that would otherwise cause us damage or make us sick. For example, we react reflexively to heat or sharp objects. Deer instinctively know to run from carnivores. Dogs bark at strangers. Animals, including humans, avoid things that smell bad, and our conscious perception of them as noxious is because they would harm us. We refuse to drink cloudy or green water, avoid eating things that don't smell good, or throw up something foul that we mistakenly ingest. These are all instinctive and learned nervous system responses that are part of our proactive immune system.

The key take-home message here is that the ANS motivates us, instinctively, to fight, flee, or avoid danger. In concert with this response is an increase in sympathetic activity (called sympathetic "tone"), causing release of norepinephrine in the brain and peripherally. Once the danger has passed and the threat no longer perceived, parasympathetic tone rises and there is a release of acetylcholine. This corresponds with the release of pent-up energy and entering into a rest, digest, recover, and restore mode. The importance of acetylcholine release goes to the core of this book. But before we can get there, we need to explain a few more players in this incredibly important story.

MITOCHONDRIA

Turning back to eukaryote cells, whether they are single-celled amoeba or the endothelial lining cells in an elephant's digestive tract, all have a common feature that is quite literally the reason for their existence: mitochondria. In fact, we could divide prokaryotes from eukaryotes, not based on the presence of a nucleus, but whether the cell contains mitochondria. That is, all cells that have a nucleus have mitochondria, almost certainly because organelles would not be possible without the energy provided by mitochondria.

Life arose on the planet Earth nearly four billion years ago. In fact, given the violence of those early epochs, it is likely that life arose, was decimated, and arose again, repeatedly. For more than a billion years these early lifeforms survived in an environment with virtually no free oxygen, often harnessing reactions involving hydrogen sulfide as the energy drivers for their life-sustaining biochemistry. About 2.8 billion years ago, however, an emergent class of these ancient single-celled animals, called cyanobacteria (blue-green algae), took over the oceans and literally transformed the atmosphere, lifting the oxygen concentration to a remarkable 2 percent (still measly by modern standards).

The arrival of highly reactive oxygen in the atmosphere was toxic to many of the anaerobic bacteria. In this environment, the ability to use the new "potent pollutant" to generate energy was an incredible advantage. The ancestors of mitochondria were these upstart lifeforms. The endosymbiotic origin theory suggests that a merger of two cells, one being an old anaerobe and the other being the ancestor of the modern mitochondria, joined forces around 2.5 billion years ago, leveraging the value of size and strength (the anaerobe) with prodigious energy production capacity and oxygen tolerance (the mitochondria).

In financial terms, this was the greatest merger of all time. Mitochondria provided nearly limitless investment capital (energy) for research and development, enabling new organelle structures along with new and innovative ways to store, copy, deploy, and use genetic material. Expansion was inevitable, and the host cells became larger and more capable. As they did, the number of mitochondria within each one grew. For example, a human egg cell, from which an entire person is constructed, contains an estimated 500,000 mitochondria. Hepatocytes (liver cells) can have up to 20 percent of their volume filled with one to two thousand mitochondria. Human heart cells (cardiomyocytes) are 40 percent mitochondria. The muscles controlling the wings of a hummingbird are similarly stacked with mitochondria, and their mitochondria have substantially more capacity to generate energy.

Internal changes made possible by mitochondria led to inter-cellular communications and more profound partnerships within communities of cells. These partnerships became formalized, and multicellular lifeforms with cellular specialization arose. The explosion of land, sea, and airborne animals, as well as trees, grasses, and flowering plants, owe their existence to this merger.

As these milestones in evolution were reached, the partnership itself was adjusted, with most genetic material from the mitochondria migrating to the nucleus of the host cell. In most advanced animals, only thirteen genes for critical proteins remain in the mitochondria, where they are copied and converted into proteins in a manner that is reminiscent of a much more primitive history. In fact, the reason that mitochondria maintain any genetic information of their own appears to be to manage certain critical features of energy generation specific for itself.

Although volumes have been written on the various functions of mitochondria, we only need to understand how healthy mitochondria generate energetic molecules that make life go, and how breakdowns in mitochondrial health can damage the health of the host. With respect to the former, recall that most biochemical reaction pathways required for life are energetically unfavorable. All cells have, therefore, evolved mechanisms to harness certain simple reactions to drive the incredible diversity of activity of which it is capable.

The most important of these reactions is simply written as ATP → ADP, where ATP stands for *adenosine triphosphate* and ADP is *adenosine diphosphate*. Structurally, both are molecules that include adenosine (an analog of the nucleic acid adenine). As their names suggest, ATP has three phosphate groups attached to it, and ADP has only two. (There is also an AMP, or adenosine monophosphate, which plays important signaling roles, often related to the failure of ATP generation.) ATP, ADP, and AMP are effectively the rechargeable batteries of cellular tools.

The production of ATP generally occurs through one of two methods. The first is very simple, and it is called glycolysis, which literally means "splitting glucose." It doesn't require oxygen (and doesn't generate carbon dioxide) and is thus described as anaerobic. It's been around since the dawn of life, and it is used by prokaryotes and eukaryotes. It is very limited in its ability to extract the energy in glucose; i.e., its waste products still contain the vast majority of the energy.

The second and far more complicated way to produce ATP is through oxidative phosphorylation, which is what mitochondria do. Mitochondria use the waste and, through a multistep process that involves a host of specialized molecules and proteins, generate eighteen times the ATP that glycolysis can. In short, the mitochondria are structured like hydrogen battery cells. They pump electrons into an internal region that holds them away from the protons of hydrogen atoms. This process is referred to as the electron transport chain, or ETC, and under healthy circumstances, the current of the organic battery is only allowed to flow through a specialized protein structure that some refer to as the world's smallest machine, called ATP synthase. The flow of electrons through this protein literally turns a wheel that attaches a phosphate group to ADP, making ATP. The by-products of this electron flow are carbon dioxide and water. The role of oxygen in enabling this entire process to result in the phosphorylation of ADP to ATP is why it is referred to as oxidative phosphorylation (often abbreviated OXPHOS).

OXPHOS is a much more efficient process and produces more than thirty ATP from the waste left over from splitting a single glucose molecule. It is no wonder that the ancestors of the eukaryotes decided to internalize and keep, versus simply digesting away, their mitochondria. The additional energy enabled the specialization of cells that makes complex life-forms, like humans, possible.

MACROPHAGES

One of these exquisitely specialized cells, present in nearly all multicellular animals, was discovered a little over 120 years ago by a Russian scientist by the name of Élie Metchnikoff. Metchnikoff watched the torment of activity that arose from embedding tangerine thorns into the embryo of a starfish. The swarm of cells that swept in, crawling all over the thorns, trying to engulf and destroy them, were named macrophages because they were clearly big eaters.

Metchnikoff postulated that these macrophages were part of an immune response, designed to swallow up and digest away dangerous foreign objects. To this point in history, there were competing theories of immunity: the humoral and the cellular theories. The former claimed that chemicals in the blood are responsible for destroying pathogens, and the latter claimed that dedicated cells eradicate threats and heal the body. Of course, both sides were right. There are antibodies and other circulating factors released by cells to kill invaders. On the other hand, Metchnikoff's macrophages, along with other cells, are capable of fighting pathogens on the front lines. Metchnikoff won his Nobel Prize in 1908 for proving the cellular theory, side by side with Paul Ehrlich, who won for his work proving aspects of humoral immunity.

Metchnikoff's discovery was remarkable, but the specific experiment in which he first observed them was unfortunate. That is because macrophage function was subsequently viewed as primarily to attack and destroy things. Although they exist in nearly every nook and cranny of complex lifeforms, for generations, macrophages were viewed as cells that laid in wait, like snipers, waiting to rain violence on pathogens. To this day, for many in healthcare, this remains the prevailing opinion. Nothing could be further from the truth.

In fact, there may be no more important, and nearly omnipotent, cell in the human body than the macrophage. To understand why this is no hyperbole, we must step back to the earliest stages of gestational development. Just after its implantation in the wall of the uterus, a group of macrophages called *Hofbauer cells* pass from the placental ball and into the uterine wall of the mother. Like a land developer who must first deploy representatives to city hall to secure building permits, and then must have his or her crew cut a road to the property for supply deliveries, Hofbauer cells act as placental emissaries. They accomplish these tasks by releasing anti-inflammatory cytokines that render the maternal (decidual) macrophages docile.

Simultaneously, they release growth factors that initiate blood vessel development (angiogenesis) that will enable delivery of nutrients to the placenta as the embryo develops.

At this early point in gestation, two structures exist within the placenta (the "work zone" of the construction project). The first is the embryo, although it is not much more than three layers of cells that have a little structure beyond a rough orientation that assigns where the head and feet will be relative to one another. In a sense, this early embryonic stage is like the developer's plot of land that has been cleared and staked out, but no real building has yet taken place. The other structure within the early placenta is the yolk sac, and like the mobile home developers often transport to their building site, it is the location of a lot of early coordination and planning.

In fact, on what is referred to as embryonic day 7.5,* there is an emigration of cells from the yolk sac into four locations of the tiny embryo. This first wave is composed of macrophage progenitor cells that take up residency in the neural tube (where the brain will be built), the chest (where the heart will be), the abdomen (where the liver will be), and the dermal layer (which will become the skin). These progenitor cells proliferate and differentiate into macrophages by the hundreds, then thousands,

_____

* Similar stages of development of a fetus occur at different rates for various species, but they are roughly proportional to the overall gestational length. For ease of reference, these stages are labeled corresponding to the development day of a mouse embryo. Thus, the term embryonic day 7.5 does not actually refer to events taking place 7.5 days from conception in humans, but rather to the point in the development process for a human that mirrors what a mouse embryo is going through at that time.

then millions, and ultimately, by the billions, becoming the tissue-resident macrophage of the brain (microglia), heart (cardiac macrophages), liver (Kupffer cells), and skin (Langerhans cells). Every subsequent tissue that is created, from the kidneys and lungs to bones and reproductive organs, each has its own subclasses of tissue-resident macrophages.

As we will see in the subsequent chapters, there is no tissue in the body that does not owe its existence, maintenance, regeneration, and ultimately its senescence and demise to the tissue-resident macrophage.

If these roles were not remarkable enough, the macrophages that construct, remodel, maintain, dismantle, and regenerate every tissue in the body also have the ability to carry out critical tasks of the cells they shepherd. Examples of this include alveolar macrophages in the lung that have been shown to transform themselves into nerve cells and literally synapse with other nerves and to release neurotransmitters in order to transmit pain signals. Kupffer cells have been observed transporting and storing iron the way hepatocytes do in times of liver injury or dysfunction.

In the coming chapters, where the roles of the nervous system, the immune system, and mitochondria are discussed with respect to development, optimization, pathologies, and degeneration of the brain, metabolic systems, and reproductive systems, the specific roles of the tissue-resident macrophages will be crucial.

THE IMMUNE REFLEX

Nearly a quarter century ago, a discovery was made that turned the fields of immunology, rheumatology, and neurology on their collective heads. When the full story of this discovery, and its consequences, is finally written, there is unlikely to be a single field of medicine, from obstetrics to oncology, and from pediatrics to geriatrics, that won't have been utterly transformed. For now, let's start at the beginning.

As with all major discoveries, there were hints that preceded the major leap forward by decades. For example, French and British surgeons of the 1930s and 1940s had removed the spleens of rheumatoid arthritis patients with some remarkable success. Also, in the late 1960s, Russian scientists had found that cutting the vagus nerve, the primary component of the parasympathetic arm of the ANS, prior to triggering a severe allergic reaction could keep an animal from dying from anaphylactic shock. The former revealed the role of the spleen in pathological inflammatory responses, and the latter demonstrated that the ANS was linked to the pathological immune reactions.

The quantum leap forward came in 2000 when Luydmila Borovikova and colleagues, working under the direction of Dr. Kevin Tracey at the Feinstein Institute on Long Island, New York, published a letter to *Nature*, one of the leading journals in all of science.[3] At the time (the late 1990s), the Feinstein Institute team was studying a polypeptide with the code name CNI-1493 and its effects on severe immune reactions, such as those that occur with septic shock. Shock is a life-threatening condition, typically triggered by infective agents (viral or bacterial) and involving the release of overwhelming quantities of inflammatory cytokines (the chemical mediators of the immune system). Septic shock is a relatively common and serious problem, with more than 1.7 million cases in the United States annually and contributing to more than a quarter of a million deaths.

The team at the Feinstein Institute had been studying a model of septic shock that involves injecting a molecule called lipo-polysaccharide, or LPS, that is found in the cell membrane of certain prokaryotes into rodents. As previously mentioned, some of the cell membrane components of prokaryotes, including LPS, are robust triggers of the immune system, triggering production of inflammatory cytokines. It is the overwhelming production of these cytokines that leads to the clinical symptoms of sepsis.

In these studies, CNI-1493 (also known as semapimod) was injected in relatively large quantities into the peritoneum (non-organ regions within the abdomen), and it was observed to reduce the expression of inflammatory cytokines. After observing these results, Kevin Tracey injected minute quantities of semapimod into the cerebral spinal fluid–filled regions of the brains of some of the animals. To his surprise, he found that these tiny quantities were able to arrest the inflammatory cytokine release as effectively as large amounts introduced into the peritoneum. To him, this suggested that the effects of the polypeptide treatment might involve the nervous system. An investigation into this possibility led to the discovery that semapimod was activating an area of the brain called the dorsal motor nucleus of the vagus nerve. Armed with this observation, the Feinstein Institute team decided to test whether electrical stimulation of the vagus nerve might also be able to affect the severity of a septic response.*

In the study cited above, the Feinstein Institute team divided a collection of normal rats into four groups. The first group was used as a control, and levels of their inflammatory cytokines were measured to be negligible. The second group was injected with LPS and, predictably, generated severe inflammatory responses, with sharp increases in cytokine expression. The third group of animals had LPS administered to them, but they also had their vagus nerves cut, and an even higher level of cytokine release was measured.** The study authors explained these results by stating that cutting the vagus nerve released the natural braking mechanisms that exist to resist significant cytokine expression. The final group of animals in the experiment mirrored the third group, except, after cutting the vagus nerve, the researchers electrically stimulated the exposed ends of the nerve. The results were astounding. The levels of cytokine expression in these animals were suppressed by nearly 90 percent.

Over the ensuing years, many research teams around the world have contributed to the description of the pathway(s) by which this vagus nerve stimulation (VNS) suppresses cytokine expression.[4] It goes something like this:

---

* Although the work in anaphylaxis and asthma that our team developed, starting in 2005, was done without knowledge of the Feinstein Institute team's work, there is no debating that their work preceded ours.

** This is the one finding that has been challenged by subsequent researchers, and it appears to be the one variable response that is not consistently reproduceable.

The vagus nerve interacts with the splenic nerve, a sympathetic nerve, at the celiac plexus. VNS activates the splenic nerve to fire, releasing norepinephrine into the spleen. This norepinephrine release activates a special set of T-cells, called ChAT+ cells, that respond to norepinephrine release by releasing acetylcholine. This release of a neurotransmitter by an immune cell in response to a neurotransmitter is a wonderful demonstration of how the immune system and the nervous system are really two sides of the same coin. The acetylcholine binds a special receptor on the surfaces of macrophages within the spleen, as well as circulating monocytes traveling through the spleen, referred to as the alpha-7 nicotinic acetylcholine receptor, or α7-nAChR. Binding of acetylcholine to this receptor causes multiple separate pathways to activate, each of which has anti-inflammatory effects. An important function of several of these pathways is to block nuclear factor kappa-light-chain-enhancer of activated B cells, thankfully abbreviated NF-κB, which would otherwise activate the expression of many genes associated with inflammation.

It should be noted that subsequent work has shown that stimulating the ends of the cut vagus nerves that still connect to the brain can also activate this pathway. Other authors have suggested that this central pathway may involve signals traveling down the sympathetic chain directly to the splenic nerve from the brain. The possibility that there may be multiple ways to trigger this mechanism demonstrates that it is very robust. The existence of the pathway in nearly every complex animal in which it has been studied suggests that evolution has preserved it as critical.

Subsequent to the discovery of the splenic pathway, now referred to as the splenic cholinergic anti-inflammatory pathway, or CAP, researchers discovered that the same stimulation parameters also activated areas of the brain that lead to central acetylcholine release.[5] The importance of this observation can't be overstated. This brain-CAP has similar anti-inflammatory effects, affecting microglia (the tissue-resident macrophages of the brain) just as acetylcholine release in the spleen affected splenic macrophages. As will be seen in the next chapter, this may explain the efficacy of VNS in epilepsy, depression, and migraine, where the therapy is already approved, as well as the promise it holds for the treatment of conditions ranging from autism spectrum disorder and schizophrenia to PTSD, traumatic brain injury, stroke, and even Parkinson's and Alzheimer's disease. Here is a synopsis of how the CAP works in the brain:

> VNS causes a signal to enter the brainstem through a structure called the nucleus tractus solitarius, or NTS. The NTS contains some very important structures that release specific neurotransmitters. These include the locus coeruleus, or LC, that is the brain's sole source of norepinephrine. Adjacent to the LC is the dorsal raphe nucleus, or DRN, which is a major source of serotonin for the brain, and is activated when the LC is activated. After the LC and the DRN, another critical area, called the nucleus basalis of Meynert, or the NBM, is activated. The NBM is the brain's primary source of acetylcholine, and when it is activated by VNS, it releases acetylcholine both synaptically (as a result of nerves firing) and constitutively (a constant general dispersion throughout the brain caused by intentional leakage from specific points along the axon of the nerves).

Just as the macrophages of the spleen have α7-nAChRs on their surfaces, so do microglia (the tissue-resident macrophages of the brain).

In 2012, a team of Ukrainian researchers, led by Dr. Marina Skok, published a paper[6] that added a profound additional dimension to the cholinergic anti-inflammatory pathway when they disclosed that mitochondria express the same 7-nACh receptor.[*] Their subsequent work, confirmed by Kevin Tracey's team in 2014[7] and others, showed that acetylcholine released by VNS prevents the release of mitochondrial DNA that can trigger potent inflammatory signaling within the cell as well as the regulation of hole formation in the mitochondrial membrane and the leakage of contents that activate cell suicide (apoptosis).

Understanding the roles of the autonomic nervous system in regulating immune function (whether VNS to reduce inflammation and macrophage behavior, or sympathetic activation that enhances inflammatory signaling) is both a remarkable revelation for understanding how life operates, as well as a powerful mechanism to harness for therapeutic purposes.

---

[*]   The first published evidence of mitochondrial expression of α7-nAChRs actually comes from work done in 1984 (R. J. Lukas, "Detection of Low-Affinity Alpha-Bungarotoxin Binding Sites in the Rat Central Nervous System," *Biochemistry* 23, no. 6 [1984]: 1160–1164).

CHAPTER 2

. . . .

THE BRAIN

Any list of the biggest unsolved mysteries in science must include the so-called Hard Problem of Consciousness. In a nutshell, the Problem can be summed up as "providing the rules and requirements for a physical system to be considered conscious." Notwithstanding Aristotle's belief that the brain was merely a radiator and that the heart did the cognitive lifting for humans, it has been widely believed for millennia that processing of sensory information occurs in the brain.

The greatest philosophers and scientists in human history, from Hippocrates, Plato, and Galen to René Descartes and Isaac Newton, struggled with the question of how interactions of light, sound, chemicals, and physical objects with our sense organs could give rise to thought and perception. While Descartes proposed (without any evidence) that the pineal gland was the locus connecting the physical tissue and an ethereal world of perceptions, it has only been within the last century that discoveries relating to synapses, neurotransmitters, ion channels (coupled to receptors or otherwise), fast and slow transmission mechanisms, and reuptake pathways helped reveal the basics of how neurons function.

More recently, the development of artificial neural networks, many of which have turned out to function in much the same way as important structures in our brains do, has also advanced our understanding of the central nervous system. Still, there is something missing. The human brain has approximately 86 billion neurons and over 100 trillion synapses. By comparison, ChatGPT (GPT-4), has 175 billion artificial neurons (nodes in the multilayer transformer network) and 100 trillion connections, which, at least numerically, matches or exceeds the human brain. It is a remarkable piece of machinery, but anyone who has interacted with it long enough will certainly recognize that it is not the equivalent of a human intellect. That is, despite its ability to produce a graduate-level term paper in fractions of a second, and even its ability to report that it "enjoyed" writing the treatise, it utterly lacks the characteristics necessary to be considered conscious and have the breadth of general intelligence that a human brain does.

To understand why that is, it is important to understand how the brain develops.

MICROGLIA AND NEURODEVELOPMENT

Along with its 86 billion neurons, the brain comprises many other cells that are intricately intertwined and interact with neurons and one another. The largest three classes of cells are astrocytes, oligodendrocytes, and microglia. The first of these cell types to be studied were the electrically firing variety, the neurons. Astrocytes and oligodendrocytes, which wrap themselves around the synapses and blood vessels, and long axons, respectively, were both found to be support cells for neuronal function.

Microglia, the smallest of these "other cells," were initially referred to as glue for the network (the name actually means "little nerve glue"). Actually, as stated in chapter 1, microglia are not glue; they are the resident macrophages of the brain. Over the past few decades, however, as the amazing roles played by these cells have been deciphered, they are turning the entire view of how brains work on its, well, head. Neurons may be the wires of the neural network, but microglia are the engineers and maintenance crews that design and execute the What, Where, When, How, and Why of brain organization and function.

Like any superheroes, microglia have a compelling origin story. As introduced in chapter 1, the story of microglia begins just a few days after conception, when the first wave of macrophage progenitor cells flows from the yolk sac into the tiny embryo.[8] Extending the prior analogy of the construction site, this wave of macrophages is like the subcontractors leaving the builder's mobile home, heading into the scaffolding to begin building a 100-story office building. The first ones to arrive are the iron worker* (the liver), the plumbers (the heart), the sheetrockers, framers, and roofers (the skin), and the electricians (the brain). When the electrical subcontractors arrive on a raw site, they have to start from scratch, building wiring harnesses, conduits, and switches as much as they are laying wires and connecting outlets. Microglia also have to start from scratch.

Starting from scratch means that microglia build the entire network of neurons connected to other neurons. More specifically, microglia recruit stem cells, guide their differentiation,

---

* Do you get it? The liver is filled with iron and has a huge role in iron metabolism throughout the body. I thought that was a good pun ... but I'm a Dad, and my kids cringe and shake their heads at my jokes.

and promote neural progenitor cells to produce neurons by the billions, and then instruct each newly formed neuron where to migrate and how to terminally differentiate (e.g., into excitatory or inhibitory neurons). Just as they are promoting the growth of new neurons, the microglia also gobble up and recycle these neurons (and even their progenitors) when they don't do what, or go where, they are told.[9]

Neurons that are deemed worthy are then hooked up together by microglia.[10] Initially, these connections, synapses, appear to be an endless random tangle. In fact, there are basic but powerful rules of organization (beyond the scope of this book), but specific instructions for 100 trillion connections in three dimensions simply do not exist. Thus, synaptogenesis occurs robustly, over-connecting the entire network throughout the latter stages of gestational neurodevelopment. In the case of human beings, this synaptogenesis continues in earnest through the first few years of life. Buried within this overconnected system, however, there is potential organization and efficiency waiting to be revealed.

Like the sculptor mounding handfuls of clay onto a pedestal prior to carving and shaping it to find the desired form buried within, microglia over-connect the network and then begin a process of synaptic pruning to reveal the desired outcome. The final product is initially unrecognizable, but slowly comes into reality as the excess material is removed.

One example of over-connectivity can be simple redundancy, such as when axons initially connect the retinae from both eyes to both the left and right optic nerves.[11] This produces double images that are not stereoscopic. Sensory data guides the microglia to prune away the right retina's synapses with the optic nerve on the left, and vice versa. This sensory-dependent pruning is tremendously important, but also dangerous. A young animal prevented from experiencing any visual stimuli during the period when the microglia are pruning the inappropriate connections will have the needed synapses also removed because sensory information isn't available to guide the pruning. This sensory-guided pruning is the will of the sculptor, and the microglia are the sculptor's hands.

In order to optimize the network for the specific demands of the environment and the animal's life, microglia gobble up and remove synapses (through a process called *trogocytosis*) so extensively, that by age fifteen, in humans, the density of synapses has dropped by 50 percent. This activity and sensory-dependent pruning also explains how intellectual stimulation as a child can literally enhance the cognitive capacity, and why we encourage the elderly to continue using their minds to prevent the loss of function and dementia.

Just as synapses can be pruned away, microglia can reinforce connections through a process referred to as long-term potentiation, or LTP. LTP is used to lower the amount of excitatory neurotransmitter necessary to activate a useful and frequently used pathway. For reasons discussed later in this chapter, overuse of excitatory neurotransmitters can cause toxic reactions that damage and even destroy neurons, so LTP serves a very important role in the good hygiene of the network.[12]

In addition to the neurogenic and synaptogenic functions, microglia also carve the network of tunnels that will become the blood vessels, recruiting and directing the progenitors of endothelial cells that will line the tunnels, and connecting the newly formed conduits to the established blood supply (i.e., the supply lines for oxygen and nutrients for the construction project). In a manner that is highly reminiscent of the development of the neural network, during the growth or regeneration phase of blood vessel development, more vessels are generated than necessary, and with more connections to established blood lines than needed.[13] Microglia then observe the flow of blood through the network of pipes they have created, and prune the dysfunctional ones from the network of conduits, and enlarge and strengthen the ones that function well. In this way, the locations of large vessels are generally common among most humans, the result of a developmental convergence driven by efficiency and function, while smaller vessels are seemingly dispersed randomly. In a sense, the construction of the neurovasculature and the synaptic network of the brain involve the same sculpting program: form follows function, producing a convergence from chaos.

This same bioarchitectural style can be seen in the creation of many organs and tissue, from the kidneys to lungs, the liver to the pancreas, and even to the trabecular structure of bone. An initial structural form is overbuilt and inefficient, followed by the superfluous being removed.

The molecular signals that guide these pruning and/or reinforcement processes are mediated by special proteins that fall into four categories: "find me" (signals that promote microglial interaction); "eat me" (signals to promote microglia to engulf and remove); "don't eat me" (signals that promote support; e.g., vessel enlargement and LTP); and "help me."[14]

Whether it is rogue neurons, inactive synapses, or dysfunctional micro-vessels, the "eat me" signals elicit pruning and the cellular debris clearance functions of microglia. All tissue-resident macrophages have this debris-clearance mode in which they engulf and digest away dead cells and other unnecessary structures. The removal of dead cells in this manner is called *efferocytosis*, and it is not inflammatory.[15] In fact, while clearing the debris, tissue-resident macrophages often are simultaneously releasing pro-growth and progenitor stimulating factors to trigger the replacement of the very cells it is clearing.

Microglial remodeling is the mechanism by which learning, memory formation, and efficient recall of previously learned information are coordinated. In a sense, microglial synaptic reinforcement and pruning activities explain the uniqueness of individual thought and perception. In this way, we are shaped by nature and nurture. Microglia prune or promote synapses in response to sensory inputs (nurture), which are inherently individual, but how they conduct this function is based on genetic factors and protein expression (nature). As we will encounter in the final chapter, our personal life experiences can alter the level of protein expression in ways that allow nurture to influence nature (epigenetics). Thus, the brain literally builds itself, pruning and promoting connections based on use in the neurological equivalent of the expression "use it or lose it." As we shall see later in the next section, failure of the microglia to prune the network correctly is an important (even critical) factor in neurodevelopmental conditions like schizophrenia (too much pruning) and autism (too little pruning).[16]

The development of the brain as described above leads to the maturation of many areas that do not significantly change once they have undergone the optimization of pruning. These include areas that control autonomic functions like heart contractions, breathing, and swallowing, all of which are largely complete before birth. Vision (typically within the first few weeks of life) and hearing (within the first six to twelve months) are areas that are also largely complete by very early in life. Other areas, like those involved in motor control and learning a new language, remain open to some greater degree of remodeling into adulthood and even old age. However, as humans age, the ability to remodel the network becomes more difficult. For example, becoming fluent in a new foreign language or learning to play new sports (especially ones requiring significant balance, like riding a bicycle or skateboard) is extremely difficult.

Of course, learning new scientific concepts, becoming familiar with new surroundings, gaining familiarity with new technologies, and a myriad of other intellectual tasks are possible at any time in a healthy human's life. There is evidence that there are areas of the brain where the steps of creating new neurons, having them migrate into proper position, connecting them (with synapses) into the established network with lots of connections, and then subjecting these new synapses to a pruning process to ensure functionality, happens throughout life. The hippocampus is a very important one of these areas, which is involved in memory formation and learning. In order for this to happen throughout life, microglia have to remain in a state where they can keep conducting and managing all the housekeeping tasks necessary to make it all possible.[17]

Murphy's Law tells us that if something can go wrong, it does go wrong. If you are anything like me, you are probably wondering what happens when the microglia stop doing their critical tasks. And if that can happen, what could make them stop doing these all-important housekeeping tasks?

Microglia are immune cells, which means they are also responsible for defending and healing the brain when trouble arises in the form of pathogens, hypoxia, trauma, or any form of stress. When trouble occurs, it is sensed through chemical signals called DAMPs and PAMPs,* and microglia move into inflammation mode. In this state, they stop doing the housekeeping tasks. If the trouble is mild and/or brief, healthy normal microglia can shift back into their housekeeping mode easily and catch up. The more severe or chronic the problem, the longer the microglia feel that they have to stay in their inflamed state. This is a key driver of symptoms, including pain, low mood, anxiety, sleep challenges, and even cognitive dysfunction (brain fog) and seizure. Without the oversight of microglia, the brain has problems reaching or maintaining normal function. If microglia are forced to remain inflammatory for long enough, however, they can lose the ability to fully return to their housekeeping functions. In these cases, the brain starts to function abnormally. This can mean that the symptoms listed above (and others) persist even in the absence of observable inflammation. Over time, the neural network itself can start to break down and degenerate.[18]

As we begin to discuss the specifics of given medical conditions, it is important to remember that microglial inflammation can arise from inflammation that is inside the brain, like trauma or pathogens, as well as outside the brain, including metainflammation associated with aging and obesity.[19]

---

* DAMPs are Damage-Associated Molecular Patterns, and PAMPs are Pathogen-Associated Molecular Patterns.

DYSFUNCTIONS OF NEURODEVELOPMENT

The exposure of expectant mothers to proinflammatory challenges, or illnesses, trauma, or even extreme stressors, activates and distracts *in utero* fetal microglia from their normal neurodevelopmental tasks. If severe enough, they can permanently alter, or prime, the unborn child's microglia in a way that makes them react to future challenges in abnormal ways. Altered microglial function can lead to greater or less susceptibility to future inflammation shifts, and it can significantly affect synaptogenesis and synaptic pruning.[20]

With respect to in utero effects, studies have demonstrated that exposing female animals to strong triggers of inflammation, such as LPS, polyinosinic:polycytidylic acid (poly I:C), significant obesity, and even severe sleep disruption, during the earliest stages of pregnancy, alters the neurodevelopment orchestrated by microglia. The laboratory of Professor Marie-Ève Tremblay at the University of Victoria in British Columbia has studied these animal models extensively, describing the dysfunctional behavior and biochemistry of altered microglia. They have cataloged how microglial dysfunction leads to disrupted structural development at a large scale, altered synaptogenesis, and aggressive pruning that, together, lead to reduced connectivity between various regions of the brain and a reduced density of synapses. These are pathological features observed in schizophrenia patients.[21]

Animal models with this pathology also exhibit parallel behaviors to human schizophrenia, including socialization difficulty, learning challenges, and incorrect processing of sensory input.

Epidemiological studies have shown correlations between prenatal maternal infections and schizophrenia in human offspring. Investigations of cytokine expression within the central nervous system (CNS) show higher levels of inflammatory signaling, consistent with microglia that are primed and/or dysfunctional. Specifically, in 2010, Alan Brown and Elena Derkits published a paper showing the effects of maternal infections on subsequent schizophrenia in the children. Their conclusion was simple: "Prenatal exposure to infection plays a role in the etiology of schizophrenia." A similar 2014 study authored by Canetta and colleagues[22] investigated the histories of nearly eight hundred schizophrenia patients, along with matched controls, for whom maternal C-reactive protein* measurements were taken during pregnancy. This study showed a statistically significant elevated risk of schizophrenia associated with maternal immune activation. Most interestingly, microglia examined from the brains of schizophrenic individuals show the altered morphology and color-associated inflammation (and dysfunctional mitochondria).

Professor Tremblay and her team have also characterized animal models of microglial dysfunction in later stages of in utero neurodevelopment.[23] In this version of the model, the consequences appear different. (The human parallel appears to be late gestation through early postnatal years; i.e., third

---

* C-reactive protein, or CRP, is a molecule made in the liver during inflammatory events. Its presence in circulation, and more specifically its elevation above a baseline level, is associated with acute and chronic inflammation. Elevated CRP is associated with many medical conditions, ranging from obesity and metabolic inflammation to cancer and heart disease. In the current context of neurodevelopmental dysfunction, the presence of elevated CRP is a surrogate for elevated inflammation.

trimester of pregnancy through about age five.) Microglial dysfunction triggered at this stage exhibits inadequate synaptic pruning, leaving a correspondingly higher density, or over-connected network of synapses. Cognitive and learning difficulties that are similar to those in schizophrenia (although interestingly, sometimes even more disabling) are present in the offspring of these animal models. The other pathological features, however, more closely align with autism spectrum disorder (ASD). That is, excessive connectivity caused by insufficient pruning leads to an inability to filter out or to suppress neural activity, which are hallmarks of autism.

Evidence of this, or similar, pathology driving ASD in humans is strong. A 2010 study published by Atladóttir and colleagues studied ten thousand diagnoses of autism among 1.6 million Danish births. The study revealed that maternal viral and bacterial infections were associated with higher rates of ASD. Similarly, a 2021 paper by López-Aranda reported on a data analysis of 150 million Americans, including more than 3.5 million children.[24] They identified a significant association between ASD diagnoses, especially among boys, subsequent to hospitalizations for infections during the first four years of life. It appears that strong immune activation, either in utero (maternal immune activation [MIA]) or during early childhood, raises the risk of ASD, especially in males.

Bipolar disorder and attention deficit hyperactivity disorder (ADHD) are also neurodevelopmental disorders, and both have also been associated with maternal immune activation. In 2013, Alan Brown and his colleagues published findings of an epidemiological study spanning the large group of bipolar depression patients whose family histories were also available within the Kaiser Permanente system in California.[25] That study revealed that bipolar disorder was nearly four times more likely to occur among the adult children of mothers who suffered with influenza during pregnancy than among expectant mothers who had not contracted the viral infection.

Similarly, over the past several years, multiple studies have been reported in the literature showing that ADHD is more likely in children of mothers with autoimmune, autoinflammatory, and metabolic inflammatory conditions like obesity and diabetes. Specifically, in 2021, Nielsen and colleagues reported the results of a cohort of over 63,000 children. They found significantly higher rates of ADHD among the children whose mothers had type 1 diabetes, any autoimmune disease (including rheumatic disorders and psoriasis), and hyperthyroidism. This study followed on the findings of a 2017 study reported by Instances and others[26] comparing among more than half a million ADHD medication users to a control group of over fifty million. They found that offspring with ADHD were more likely to have mothers with central nervous system and peripheral autoimmune diseases (e.g., multiple sclerosis and rheumatoid arthritis), type 1 diabetes, asthma, and hypothyroidism. Interestingly, these findings were virtually unchanged when typical cofactors, like infant birth weight and premature delivery, were taken into consideration, nor did it change with diagnoses of ADHD in a parent.

In 2019, Dunn and colleagues conducted an analysis of ADHD and the possible cause underlying the disease. In their words:

> Prenatal exposure to inflammation is associated with changes in offspring brain development including reductions in cortical gray matter volume and the volume of

certain cortical areas—parallel to observations associated with ADHD. Alterations in neurotransmitter systems, including the dopaminergic, serotonergic, and glutamatergic systems, are observed in ADHD populations. Animal models provide strong evidence that the development and function of these neurotransmitters' systems are sensitive to exposure to in utero inflammation. In summary, accumulating evidence from human studies and animal models, while still incomplete, support a potential role for neuroinflammation in the pathophysiology of ADHD.[27]

Taking a quick inventory of the evolving picture of neurodevelopment, the roles of the microglia are numerous and important. They infiltrate the central nervous system before it can even be called a nervous system. They take a leading role in every step of building the brain, from neurogenesis and connectivity, to building the network of blood vessels, to controlling the proliferation and functioning of support cells. Their critical functions are disturbed through exposure to inflammation or proinflammatory triggers, and the resulting changes can lead to structural and connectivity changes associated with neurodevelopmental and neuropsychiatric disorders. Ensuring that microglia remain in a noninflammatory state is considered by researchers in the field to be a critically important step for proper neurodevelopment. This is true from gestation through childhood, and even through adolescence, as there is much neurodevelopment that continues through these stages of physical development.

As Paul Patterson wrote more than a decade ago, the consequences of maternal immune activation (i.e., systemic inflammation) during pregnancy strongly suggest that steps be taken to reduce inflammation.[28] The expectation is that doing so may limit the risks of in utero neurodevelopmental problems.

How can we do that?

Pharmaceutical agents, like the tetracycline class antibiotic, minocycline, which has the ability to pass through the blood brain barrier, have been shown to influence microglia to reorient them back into an anti-inflammatory state and may be beneficial. In fact, in 2019, Megumi Andoh of the University of Tokyo published a book chapter canvassing the various studies (in both animals and humans) using pharmaceutical agents that are known to have effects on microglia, and generally found that the effects in humans with autism of these agents were decreased cytokine expression, decreased repetitive behavior, hyperactivity, and irritability, as well as increased or improved social interactions and verbal communication.[29]

These are promising insights and clearly suggest there is an ongoing role for reducing microglial activation to prevent neurodevelopmental disorders. As we shall see, these potential protective therapies include drugs, like minocycline, and neuromodulation, like vagus nerve stimulation. Given that the incidence of ASD has now risen among male children to 1 in 30 births, up from 1 in 5,000 as recently as 1990, the urgency to finding a prevention is as strong as anything. Similarly, ADHD is now observed in more than seven percent of children, and (along with bipolar disorder) are at even higher rates among offspring of mothers who are obese, have hypertension, and/or are aged over forty at the time of the birth. As terrifying as these issues are, the social challenges of schizophrenia, ranging from homelessness to mass violence, is apocalyptic. The promise of therapy that could be administered safely and over an extended period of time (through the mother during pregnancy, and from birth through age five, for example) and could reduce the disruption of microglia during development clearly would be worth the effort.

Sadly, few if any studies have tested the hypothesis that anti-inflammatory therapies may be able to prevent the neurodevelopmental challenges during pregnancy or early in life. In 2023, however, Professor Tremblay's lab initiated one such study using noninvasive VNS to activate the brain-CAP as a possible protection against MIA-induced schizophrenia and ASD in her animal models. In a separate arm of this study, VNS is being applied to a cohort of offspring, to test the potential to arrest and possibly reverse the consequences of the MIA. While it is too early to tell, the results of this study certainly have the potential to be groundbreaking.

OPTIMIZATION OF NEURODEVELOPMENT

As we have just described, severe and/or chronic inflammation can alter microglial functions to cause neurodevelopmental problems. But some level of inflammation is inevitable in a normal pregnancy, and certainly young children have inflammatory challenges, from cuts and scrapes to infections (and even from the regimen of vaccinations they undergo). The natural question that arises, therefore, is "What level of inflammation and microglial distraction is tolerable and does not interfere with neurodevelopment?"

Unfortunately, the answer appears that all inflammation negatively impacts neurodevelopment. That is, every experience of inflammation leads to some distraction of microglia, and thus to some level of suboptimal neurodevelopment. Who doesn't want a higher IQ? And if not for yourself, for your children ... and if not for your children, then how about your financial advisor, lawyer, surgeon, or business partners?

There is strong evidence that at least some component of intelligence is genetic. This assumption begs the questions: "What are the genes that code for smarts?" and "What do they actually modulate?" A Chinese scientist named He Jiankui may have inadvertently conducted a trial that provided a glimpse into the inner workings, and sure enough, it has to do with controlling inflammation. In a widely criticized breach of medical scientific ethics, Jiankui and his colleagues used CRISPER technology to edit out a specific immune receptor called CCR5 in human embryos.[30]

Why did Jiankui select CCR5 as his target? Well, there are two very important things to know about CCR5. The first is that this receptor is the key that HIV uses to unlock the cellular door and gain entry into immune cells (T-cells). (Reportedly, Jiankui and his team were trying to engineer humans that were immune to HIV, which isn't quite as nefarious a goal as breeding genetically altered supergeniuses. Still, it was wildly unethical.) The second important thing to know about CCR5 is that the receptor's main purpose is to promote inflammation.

How, you are likely asking, does this relate to intelligence? It turns out that in 2016, a group of scientists published a survey study[31] in which they had deleted 140 separate genes from mice, one at a time, to find out if any had an effect on mouse intelligence. What they found was that CCR5 deletion gave the mice better memories. Memory is an important part of learning, and learning is a big part of intelligence. Follow-up investigations found that some people actually have naturally occurring CCR5 deletions, and these individuals appear to gain some benefits, including a faster recovery from strokes ... and they are smarter!

Hold on, you say? What do you mean smarter? Like the mice in the survey study, the lack of a CCR5 gene enhances memory, learning, and recall. The facts appear to support the conclusion that folks with faulty CCR5 receptors are better at school, learn challenging material more easily, remember it longer, apply it more effectively, and do better in jobs that depend more on intelligence. These benefits make them more capable of making more money, more apt to live healthier lives, and live longer. This led MIT's *Technology Review* magazine to title their 2019 article (cited above) about the Chinese experiment, "China's CRISPER twins might have had their brains inadvertently enhanced."

Again, this is all very consistent with the conclusion that inflammation, which disrupts microglia, causes neurodevelopmental inefficiencies and results in less optimal intellect.

If *any* inflammatory activation of microglia will disrupt neurodevelopment, at least to some degree, then we have *all* experienced neurodevelopment in an environment that is suboptimal. Optimizing neurodevelopment, or allowing a person to reach his or her full potential, isn't a bad thing, but even if sanctioned by an ethics review committee and demonstrated to be safe in endless animal studies, I suspect that most people would not consider genetically altering their children in utero using CRISPER technology for anything other than a lifesaving treatment. In contrast, however, even though it may sound like a plot of a *Star Trek* episode, I suspect that very few people would consider minimizing maternal inflammation during pregnancy, and for a child during early developmental years—ethically questionable.

COGNITIVE IMPROVEMENT WITH VNS

Harkening back to Professor Tremblay's ongoing study to test if VNS might positively impact neurodevelopment, is there any evidence that this therapy provides cognitive improvement? Enticingly, there is ample evidence that the answer is yes. For example, in adults with PTSD, a recent study led by Dr. Doug Bremner revealed the ability to learn and recall material at a significantly improved rate (nearly double) among a cohort using a noninvasive VNS device compared with subjects using a sham device.[32]

Similarly, studies looking at cognitive functions in patients who have received implanted VNS devices for drug-resistant depression, improvements in multiple aspects of cognitive function were reported. In one such study, Véronique Jodoin of the University of Quebec demonstrated that VNS improved learning and memory within one month of initiating treatment for depression, and the benefits were maintained for at least two years.[33]

In an interesting study that attempted to identify the ways in which VNS was exerting its cognitive enhancing effects, researchers found that the therapy enhanced connectivity between the default mode and executive networks.[34] These networks, along with the salience network that relays the information back and forth between them, are associated with creativity. These findings provide anatomical support for vagus nerve stimulation as an activator of creativity.

These prior studies were conducted in patients with depression. More recently, the study of cognitive benefits associated with VNS transitioned from a curious side effect to a primary use in healthy normal individuals. Specifically, data published by Andrew McKinley and Lindsey McIntire showed significant cognitive improvement among healthy normal volunteers who were stressed by sleep deprivation. The study revealed that noninvasive vagus nerve stimulation enabled the volunteers to answer questions correctly immediately after an initial sleep-deprived period of learning, and again days and even weeks later. Follow-on work in foreign language learning and spatial relations applications have continued to produce evidence that noninvasive vagus nerve stimulation can provide cognitive enhancement in adults.[35]

But what about children? Studies in children with epilepsy treated with implanted VNS devices have tested improved cognitive ability, including verbal ability.[36]

The data appear to be piling up that VNS, with its ability to shift microglia from an inflammatory mode back to a housekeeping state, not only reduces cognitive dysfunction associated with other medical conditions, but appears to optimize ongoing neurodevelopment in the hippocampus, improving learning and recall. In children who are undergoing massive neurodevelopment, reducing inflammation should mean optimizing neurodevelopment.

THE ADULT BRAIN

Given the description of how brains develop, it is understandable that many important functions have either been learned, or not, and therefore, are effectively baked in by adulthood. This is why you never forget how to ride a bike if you learn as a child, but learning to ride a bike as an adult is virtually impossible. Ongoing neurogenesis and synaptogenesis in key areas, like the hippocampus, however, require microglial involvement and management in the same way as in neurodevelopment. That is, neural progenitor cells cause new neurons to come into existence, regulated by the release of growth and differentiation factors, and these neurons must be directed to migrate to the appropriate locations. This migration can be challenging in the dense structure that is already present, which leads upwards of 90 percent of new neurons to be triggered to self-destruct (a process called *apoptosis*). The clearance of these dead cells is managed by microglial cells in their normal anti-inflammatory mode of debris clearance, or efferocytosis.

That is a lot of work for microglia to perform! It is, however, just the tip of the iceberg when it comes to the tasks of the microglia. Their control of inflammatory signaling influences mood, proper sleep, perceptions and responses to pain, and they manage changes in oxygenation level, the clearance of toxins, the mobilization of iron and other trace minerals, and the clearance and replacement of dysfunctional mitochondria within the neurons of the network. Microglia have a hand in nearly every activity that takes place within the brain. For obvious reasons, therefore, dysfunction among microglia can have significant negative impacts on mental and physical health.

UNDERSTANDING DEPRESSION

Major depressive disorder (MDD) and anxiety are two of the most prevalent medical conditions in the modern world. According to the National Institute for Mental Health, one in twelve adults in the US suffers with depression in a given year, and among the youngest category of eighteen to twenty-five-year-olds, the rate is more than one in six! Anxiety conditions, obsessive-compulsive disorder, and social and general anxiety disorders affect nearly 20 percent of the population of the United States annually, and a staggering 31 percent of the adult population experiences episodes of a clinically diagnosable anxiety disorder within their lifetimes. Post-traumatic stress disorder (PTSD) is its own category, and it affects another close to 5 percent of the population.[37]

From the 1950s and 1960s to today, there has been an appreciation, bordering on fixation, of the role neurotransmitter imbalances as it relates to both of these disorders. To be fair, lower levels of serotonin observed in depressed patients does mean less serotonin is released and lower levels of the neurotransmitter remain in the synapse long enough to be effective. Whether depression is caused by this lack of serotonin is debated, even today. Believers refer to this line of thinking as the Monoamine Theory,[38] and it has led to the development of classes of drugs, like monoamine oxidase inhibitors (MAOIs), tricyclic antidepressants, and selective serotonin reuptake inhibitors (SSRIs), all of which do have depression-relieving properties. This final class of drugs includes some of the most widely prescribed medications in the country, and world, including such popular brand names as Paxil, Celexa, Lexapro, Zoloft, and Prozac. All are variants based on this

Monoamine Theory, with MAOIs blocking the breakdown on neurotransmitters, and SSRIs targeting the reuptake mechanisms so that the available serotonin remains in synapse longer.

By way of background for the discussion to follow, serotonin was discovered in the context of intestinal motility, and it is often stated that 90 percent of the serotonin in the body is produced by the gut, in concert with the healthy microbiome that exists there. In fact, serotonin is produced by nearly every cell in the body, and by nearly every organism on Earth. The release of serotonin from the cell, however, either as a neurotransmitter (by neurons), a coordinator of clotting (platelets), or as a regulator of the growth of mammary glands, is reserved for specific cells. In the context of the central nervous system, serotonin is also known as the "feel good" neurotransmitter because it is involved in the maintenance of mood and the inhibition of pain signaling through one of the two primary descending inhibition pathways (in concert with GABA).[39] Medications that target the serotonin receptors associated with pain modulation (and regulation of vascular tone) include triptan medications for headache (discussed later in this chapter). And, as we discussed in the paragraph above, medications that target the reuptake mechanisms for serotonin, called reuptake inhibitors, are used to treat depression.

The trouble is that, while many of these SSRIs show efficacy for a period of time, their mood-improving benefits fade (while their side effects do not).[40] To understand why this may be the case, we need to take a deeper dive into the What, Where, How, and Why of serotonin metabolism. And as you might have guessed, the story involves microglia.

THE ROLE OF INFLAMMATION
IN SICKNESS BEHAVIOR

Microglia influence both serotonin synthesis and its reuptake mechanism, both of which are critical to the health of the brain, and can be altered by inflammation. To understand how the immune system regulates serotonin, and why, it is necessary to dive (briefly) into the chemistry of serotonin synthesis. The amino acid tryptophan is converted into serotonin through a two-step process that includes the action of two enzymes.[*] In the presence of inflammatory cytokines (including TNF-α, IL-1, and IFN-γ), the production of another enzyme called indol-amine 2,3-dioxygenase (IDO) is increased (upregulated).[41] This disrupts, or at least reduces, serotonin synthesis, which has a number of negative consequences.

What is the evolutionary rationale for having inflammation upregulate IDO? From its discovery in the 1960s until the late 1990s, it was believed that the principal benefit of IDO was in its ability to deprive tumor cells and bacteria of tryptophan. We now know that IDO helps to make the interior of the cell inhospitable (and downright hostile) to microbial and viral invaders. It does this by promoting an alternate biochemical pathway that generates free radical–promoting metabolites, including kynurenine and quinolinic acid,[42] which does use up available tryptophan, but these free radicals do a lot of damage to the cell, and the mitochondria.

---

[*] Hydroxylation by L-tryptophan hydroxylase followed by decarboxylation with L-aromatic amino acid decarboxylase. In plants, the process can proceed in opposite order.

Bringing this back around to depression, increased IDO expression means less serotonin production, and thus, not surprisingly, kynurenine and quinolinic acid are found in elevated concentrations in the cerebral spinal fluid of many patients with MDD. It is also found in higher concentrations in patients who suffer with chronic inflammation, or who have increased levels of inflammatory cytokines in circulation.[43] In part, this is the reason why depression is a comorbidity of inflammatory conditions and is often referred to as sickness behavior.

The consequences of reduced serotonin synthesis go further. Physical and mental symptoms of depression (and sickness) often include fatigue, which is tied to the energy metabolism of the cell. This effect may be related to reduced synthesis of melatonin, which plays an important role in the healthy functioning of mitochondria.[44] More specifically, melatonin is produced in a two-step biochemical reaction that uses serotonin as the principal precursor. These particulars of this role of melatonin in mitochondrial health will be addressed more fully later, after a discussion of excitotoxicity (the damage that can occur when neurons are forced to be in an excited state for too long) and some of the clinical conditions associated with that phenomenon.

Commercially available drugs that block or reduce IDO include Vioxx and Celebrex, which were designed to act at the COX-2 (cyclooxygenase-2) receptor to block inflammation. Both enhance serotonin to support the pain-reducing benefits of serotonin.

If the only effect of inflammatory cytokines was to reduce serotonin synthesis, then preventing the reuptake of the serotonin from the synapse, as SSRIs are designed to do, would make the little bit of available serotonin last longer. Unfortunately, inflammatory cytokines also upregulate the expression of the transporters that facilitate the reuptake of the serotonin.[45] That is, in the presence of TNF-α and/or IL-1, the number of serotonin transporters (SERT) that remove serotonin from the synapse get larger. In a very real sense, therefore, inflammatory cytokines are the equivalent of selective serotonin reuptake *enhancers*, working in exact opposition to SSRIs.

Given this perspective, it is no wonder that medications that reduce the inflammatory state of microglia often have mood-elevating benefits for patients with depression and anxiety. This includes minocycline, a member of the tetracycline family of antibiotics that appears to have the ability to suppress proinflammatory microglial activation, which will be discussed at various additional points in this section.

EXCITOTOXICITY

Disruption of serotonin and melatonin pathways are only two ways in which inflammatory cytokines released from acti-vated microglia can alter brain function. Before we head into a deeper conversation about melatonin, it is worth veering off on an important tangent to address another phenomenon, *exci-totoxicity*, which also involves inflammatory microglial signals that trigger neuronal problems. In a nutshell, excitotoxicity is the excessive release of glutamate and the excessive respon-siveness of the neurons to it, which can cause neuronal stress, dysfunction, and death.[46]

To understand this, recall that glutamate is the principal excit-atory neurotransmitter of the central nervous system. That means that neurons all over the brain release glutamate as a signal to activate the next neuron with which they are synapsed. Astrocytes that control the levels of neurotransmitters in the synaptic cleft convert glutamate into glutamine and return it to the pre-synaptic neuron to be turned back into glutamate for release again.

Now, proinflammatory microglia release TNF-α and other inflammatory cytokines. These cytokines can act on the same cell that released them, by binding to receptors on the cell surface, exacerbating or prolonging the cell's inflammatory activation (this is called *autocrine activation signaling*). In another example of an immune cell releasing a neurotransmitter, these activated microglia can release glutamate into the region around the synapse. This increases the excitation level of the neurons. Remember that the process of long-term potentiation (LTP) is designed to lower the amount of glutamate needed to activate neurons that are frequently activated because too much glutamate can be harmful.

The TNF-α released by microglia also alters astrocytes that are monitoring the synapse as well, by inhibiting and even reversing the glutamate uptake receptors and channels used to remove the excitatory neurotransmitter from the synapse. That means microglia force astrocytes to contribute to the over-excitation risk.

Neurons also express TNF-α receptors, and binding to them causes an upregulation in glutamate receptors (i.e., AMPA and NMDA receptors). This makes an already bad situation worse, like wearing megaphones taped to your ears at a loud rock concert. As a last line of defense against overstimulation, neurons express $GABA_A$ receptors that are inhibitory.

Tragically, but predictably, TNF-α reduces the expression of these receptors, as well.

Why is all of this important? One of the primary drivers of migraine, seizure, and even the damage done to brain tissue in the wake of a stroke is a result of this excitotoxicity phenomenon. Finding ways to decrease this impact is critical, which means reducing microglial activation and reducing inflammation. As will be described in further detail in a section or two, VNS has been approved for several of these medical conditions and is being studied in the others.

MELATONIN AND MITOCHONDRIAL HEALTH

But first, another benefit of VNS is the reduction in mental and physical fatigue. This fatigue has been correlated with increases in inflammatory cytokine production, and the reduction of the fatigue as a result of VNS correlated with a reduction in those cytokines.[47] Since fatigue is often associated with reduced mitochiondrial function, it is reasonable to wonder how inflammation affects mitochondria.

Thus, the next part of the serotonin story is melatonin and its relationship with mitochondria. As was previously mentioned, tryptophan is the precursor for serotonin. Serotonin is, in turn, the precursor for melatonin. Thus, inflammation that suppresses serotonin production also inhibits melatonin. However, while serotonin is important and deficits of it affect mood and pain (among other things), a lack of it can completely disable cellular function. Melatonin is an essential chemical for life, made by both plant and animal cells, and utilized as a key anti-oxidant that keep mitochondria safe.

To understand this, recall from chapter 1 that mitochondria are the sites for oxidative phosphorylation (OXPHOS) to generate ATP in eukaryotic cells. The energetic processes that enable OXPHOS to produces lots of ATP can also produce damaging reactive oxygen species (ROS). At first, these ROS were thought to be a collateral risk associated with the high energy processes concentrated in the mitochondrial membrane structure, but as is often the case, Mother Nature makes use of everything. Thus, more recently, ROS have been recognized to be a signaling mechanism utilized by mitochondria to communicate with the host cell. Still, ROS are damaging and need to be managed. Mitochondria produce antioxidants (as does the host cell) including superoxide dismutase and others to reduce these molecules. Melatonin is one of these, and as such it is a regulator of mitochondrial health.[48]

This becomes especially important under inflammatory conditions when the precursor of melatonin goes into short supply, a fact that is evidenced by the retention by mitochondria of the ability to generate their own melatonin (from serotonin).[49]

In the absence of sufficient antioxidant, ROS damage to mitochondrial DNA continues until it reaches a certain threshold. Coupled with calcium ion buildup, which is discussed next, the mitochondria respond by ejecting their DNA into the intracellular medium outside the mitochondria (in the cytosol). Since DNA isn't supposed to be floating around the cytosol of a eukaryotic cell, it is a potent signal of damage and/or a pathogen being present. This signal leads to the activation of a robust proinflammatory pathway known as STING[50] (which is the acronym for "stimulator of interferon genes"). Of course, even more inflammation exacerbates the melatonin shortfall.

Brief periods of serotonin and melatonin deficit can be tolerated. For the benefit of the cell's defense, however, extended periods of stress lead to a progressive accumulation of damage from ROS. This ROS-mediated damage leads to a cascade of events, including the leakage of a key compound used in OXPHOS called *cytochrome-c*. Even small releases of cytochrome-c can have follow-on effects on another organelle, the endoplasmic reticulum (ER), leading to leakage of calcium ions from it (the ER contains large calcium stores).[51] Because cytochrome-c is maintained in the mitochondria through simple electrostatic forces, excessive calcium ion release from the ER can lead to even more cytochrome-c release. You can see where this is going: there is a positive feedback loop that is making each situation progressively worse.

If not otherwise modulated, this positive feedback loop can ultimately result in the activation of a series of proteins, including caspase 9, which promote cell suicide.[52]

Understanding the role of melatonin and the effects that inflammation has on mitochondria help to explain one of the most important but otherwise inexplicable features of the inflammatory cascade, which is the fact that inflamed microglia tend to rely on glycolysis and seem to have little or no OXPHOS. As will be discussed in chapter 3, with respect to metabolic disease, when inflammatory conditions arise that stress mitochondria, glycolysis becomes the source of ATP that cells must rely on. This will lead cells to signal that they need the liver to produce excess glucose to meet the energy demands of the immune system.[53] This reliance on glycolysis means that the demand for glucose is much higher to maintain normal cellular functions and blood glucose levels rise dangerously, driving more insulin release. Symptoms of mental and physical fatigue are common among inflammatory conditions, and a significant cause is this mitochondrial dysfunction.

Now, there are two positive feedback loops that have just been described, and both are tied to the fact that inflammation is affecting melatonin production, and involving mitochondrial dysfunction. Neither appear to have a clear off-ramp from a vicious cycle. If you have been wondering how this ties back to autonomic nervous system control of inflammation, then this is the "drop the mic" moment.

Mitochondria express the α7 nicotinic acetylcholine receptor.

First, with respect to the mitochondrial DNA release that causes inflammation, binding of the α7-nAChR inhibits the release of mitochondrial DNA, delaying the trigger for the conversion of the cell to an inflammatory orientation.[54] For these reasons, the α7-nAChR is sometimes referred to as a cell survival receptor as it inhibits the cell from committing programmed cell death.

Next, regarding the calcium and cytochrome-c problem, it turns out that mitochondria have ion channels in the outer membranes called *voltage-dependent anion channel (VDAC)* to regulate the movement of calcium ions. When VDAC becomes blocked or inhibited, calcium ions flow more readily into the mitochondria, disrupting the stability of cytochrome-c, allowing it to leak out. The activation of α7-nAChR acts to restore proper function of VDAC,[55] thereby preventing the buildup of calcium ions in the mitochondria and preventing the leakage of cytochrome-c.

These mechanisms explain why VNS, which leads to a release of acetylcholine, is an important protector of cell energy production, and fights fatigue and other metabolic issues, as will be seen in the next chapter. First, however, how does all of this science translate clinically?

CHAPTER 3

CLINICAL APPLICATIONS

DEPRESSION

My father was an old-school doctor; he was not interested in sports cars or fancy homes. His one indulgence was finding the time to go on vacation somewhere warm, preferably on the water somewhere without a phone or television, to truly get away and decompress. He passed away in the fall of 2022, after a good life, and God gave him a graceful exit from this world. It was fitting, given that he had helped to safely shepherd close to six thousand healthy infants into the world, and always made sure their mothers survived the arduous process.

He trained to be a physician during an age when looking for root causes of a problem was something physicians did regularly. In those days, there was no internet to search for answers, much less AI-assisted telemedicine providers dispensing drugs based on select data presented in pharma-subsidized journals and advocated by societies run by lawyers and industry experts. It made him humble but observant and kept his memory sharp and thankful for his keen ability to identify patterns. More importantly than all of that, however, was his willingness to accept that he didn't have all the answers. His allegiances weren't to the status quo or to status symbols. He just thought about things and figured it out for himself, which, in today's conformist world, would have made him an iconoclast. When I look in the mirror, of course, I see a face that is slowly becoming my father's. With that resemblance in mind, let's tackle the subject of depression with an iconoclastic spirit.

Mood is a fluid concept. What makes a person feel down one day and happy the next? Life events certainly play a big role, but most of those feelings are emotions, distinct from mood. A person can feel down about something that has happened, but so long as the biochemistry in the brain and the behavioral responses are normal, we can consider a low mood to be normal. It's also normal to be in a foul mood if someone totaled your car. Mood, brain chemistry, and behavior deviating from what is normal, based on the circumstances of your life, is generally a much more appropriate sign of pathology. In these situations, it makes a lot of sense to look at the state of the immune system.

We have already introduced the concept of sickness behavior, and the prior sections have provided ample scientific bases for how inflammation can disrupt neurotransmitter expression and lead to mitochondrial dysfunction. At first blush, what triggers inflammation seems obvious: injuries, infections, toxins, deprivation of critically needed nutrients, and other physical insults. These are threats that require a physical intervention by the immune system cells to fight and then heal from foreign invaders and damage, respectively. (It is one of the most critical messages of this book that the fighting and healing responses cannot occur simultaneously, and remaining in fight mode, which involves sympathetic activation, for too long leads to breakdown of systems because of the reliance on the support of macrophages that get distracted when they should be returning to their housekeeping jobs under parasympathetic [vagus] control.)

Obviously, threat response mode can be triggered by physical injuries; however, why do near misses trigger inflammation? Danger avoided causes inflammatory responses, sometimes as robustly as actual injuries. Even more interestingly, the perceived threat does not even have to be one of physical harm to activate the immune system. This is because the sympathetic nervous system activation, that reacts to stressors of all types, is what activates the immune system. As intangible as psychosocial pressure, emotionally traumatic events, and even sleep deprivation may seem, the immune system is activated by them. For example, patients diagnosed with inflammatory bowel disease (an autoimmune disease), who are in remission, can be triggered to express significant increases in inflammatory cytokines by exposure to socially challenging and anxiety-provoking situations, even though there is no physical injury. Because these perceived threats can persist for extended periods of time, they are often far more damaging to mental health than a single acute physical injury.

If a nonphysical trigger can cause a shift in immune state to proinflammatory, and microglia play a vital role in neural network maintenance and ongoing development necessary for learning and memory formation, then it is time to tie these two pieces together, showing that conscious experiences and the experience of stress can shift microglial states, which alters neural function, neurotransmitter expression, and mitochondrial function.

So, taking this to the obvious conclusion: Is there evidence that depression can be alleviated by anti-inflammatory treatments?

A meta-analysis of eleven studies and over 100,000 patients, published in 2019, concluded that anti-inflammatory diet choices reduced the risk of depression, while proinflammatory diets were associated with elevated risks of depression.[56] Of course, such findings can be easily criticized for failing to take into consideration the reasons behind the adoption of one diet over another (e.g., exercise enthusiasts have lower reported rates of depression and may adopt anti-inflammatory diets for fitness reasons, leaving the antidepressant effects attributable to the exercise versus the anti-inflammatory diet).

A meta-analysis of thirty-six randomized clinical trials for anti-inflammatory medications ranging from NSAIDs and steroids to statins and diabetes medication, looking at the antidepressant effects of these medications in concert with antidepressant medications alone, was published in 2019. Based on the data found, the authors concluded, "Anti-inflammatory agents improved antidepressant treatment effects." Other meta-analyses of adjunctive use of COX-2 inhibitors and aspirin have been reported with similar positive findings compared with antidepressants alone.[57]

Of course, vagus nerve stimulation has already been approved for the treatment of medically refractory depression, and comprehensive meta-analyses of the data from multiple large randomized controlled studies with multiyear follow-up are evidence of such effects.[58]

EPILEPSY

Epilepsy is a general diagnosis referring to a number of different seizure disorders, each having a variety of different causes and seizure types (e.g., absence, petit mal, and grand mal seizures). These conditions may manifest in all ages, but often present for the first time in children. However, childhood onset seizure disorders frequently persist throughout life, and seizures can also arise in the context of trauma, systemic inflammatory conditions, and/or as a consequence of neurodegenerative conditions. (The reader may note that each of these adult-onset causes has a strong immune system connection.)

Seizure activity was recognized to be a serious pathology thousands of years ago. Ancient explanations for the causes of epilepsy were typically rooted in magic and the supernatural, often attributing seizure activity to evil spirits and demonic possession. Still, it is noteworthy that pictures of seizures were drawn on cave walls, and early humans devised a rather remarkable, albeit brutal, treatment for the condition involving bashing small holes in the skulls of epileptics, called *trepanation*. It is astounding that the survival rate from this procedure was as high as 50 percent, but even more so, the therapy must have demonstrated some level of success to have been continued.

The Roman physician, Galen, was the first to hypothesize the involvement of peripheral organs in some epileptic events based on abdominal feelings and cardiac palpitations that often precede seizures. During the Renaissance, the first recorded associations of seizures with other diseases, typically infections, were made. Modern studies have demonstrated that the risk of experiencing a seizure among those with a propensity for them is significantly enhanced during periods of serious infection and/or fever. In fact, one particularly interesting series of studies has involved injecting triggers of severe inflammation into animals with an induced propensity for seizure, and then monitoring how easily it is to trigger a seizure.[59] The conclusion of the studies is that peripheral inflammation triggers neuroinflammation and oxidative stress, and that these contribute to lowering the threshold for causing seizures. Interestingly, the area of focus for the investigators was the hippocampus, where the neural network is under constant revision and development, and they felt that inhibition of inflammation and reduction of oxidative stress had the strongest anti-seizure effects.

It was previously shown how inflammation can disrupt neurotransmitter expression (especially in the case of serotonin, although dopamine is similarly affected) and generate mitochondrial stress (through the increased level of free-radical promoter molecules and the reduction in melatonin production), and now we find that inflammation can enhance the likelihood of seizures. A natural question is whether seizures are caused by the neurotransmitter imbalance or mitochondrial dysfunction. It turns out that this question has been, and continues to be, debated, and as is often the case in such debates, both are likely part of the answer. Whatever the ultimate outcome of this controversy is, it is clear that microglia play an important role in the regulation of the brain, and their shift into an inflammatory state, temporarily, is associated with both neurotransmitter imbalance and hyperexcitation phenomena such as drive seizure. Similarly, their chronic shift into an inflammatory state can lead to metabolic dysfunction that can render seizures more likely.[60]

Researchers, including Tanya Victor and Stella Tsirka at Stony Brook University in New York, have concluded that microglial dysfunction with respect to important housekeeping tasks are instrumental in rendering the brain susceptible to initial and continued seizure activity.[61] As we have discussed, among the critical functions that microglia are programmed to carry out is neural and synaptic pruning. More specifically, seizures disrupt the normal neurogenic process in key areas of the brain, including the hippocampus. As was described earlier, the hippocampus is a region of the brain where continued neuro-genesis and synaptogenesis remain active throughout life.

As the reader may recall, neurogenesis involves a multistep process that includes the proliferation and maturation of newly created neurons (from progenitor cells), the migration of newly formed cells to their proper position, creation of connections between the newly formed neurons and the neural network into which they are being integrated, and the pruning of neurons and synapses that are not properly formed or integrated. While the signaling to promote neurogenesis is present in some forms of epilepsy, dysregulation in the migration, synaptogenesis, and pruning of the evolving network have been observed. These improperly integrated neurons, often dysfunctionally regu-lated, can form an epileptogenic center. (This association with the hippocampus may also explain the observation that cog-nitive impairment and even cognitive decline can be associated with chronic seizure disorders.)

The normal role of microglia in the clearance of improperly formed or integrated neurons and/or their synapses is supposed to be a noninflammatory process. In the case of epilepsy, however, it appears that the microglia are shifted into a proinflammatory state. This leads to the failure to integrate the new neurons properly, and as a result of the seizures, the microglia remain inflamed. The effect of this feedback system is that the inflammation is chronically heightened susceptibility to seizure. Of course, it also drives neurotransmitter imbalance and excitotoxicity.[62]

Vagus nerve stimulation was first developed to treat epilepsy, and tens of thousands of people have gained control over their condition with its regular use. Although early studies in the mechanism by which vagus nerve stimulation treats epilepsy focused on monoamine neurotransmitters,[63] studies implicating the anti-inflammatory mechanisms[64] and mitochondrial effects suggest they must be considered likely mechanisms underlying the clinical benefits of VNS.

HEADACHE

Glutamate is the brain's principle excitatory neurotransmitter, but too much expression of it, caused by inflammation, can lead to unwanted excitation. One of the consequences of that unwanted excitation can be a variety of pain conditions. Migraine is a particularly devastating one, affecting approximately 12 percent of the adult population. The problem is even worse for women, especially of childbearing years, with the number of women experiencing migraines approaching one in five. Close to two out of three women who experience migraines report their attacks coincide with their menstrual cycle.[65]

TREATING ACUTE MIGRAINES

Dr. Michael Oshinsky is a brilliant scientist at the National Institute for Neurologic Diseases and Stroke (NINDS), which is one of the twenty National Institutes for Health, where he has served as a program director for pain for nearly a decade. Before joining NINDS, he spent more than a decade at Thomas Jefferson University, where he developed a very useful animal model of migraine. It involves exposing the brains (actually the thin membrane layer, called the dura, covering the brain) of rodents to a proinflammatory mixture, the key component of which is prostaglandin.[66] When delivered for the first time, his inflammatory "soup," as he refers to it, causes a period of heightened sensitivity and painful allodynia (the experience of pain caused by light touch) for a period of hours, after which the pain resolves. Repeated administrations of the soup, once every few days for a period of thirty days, however, leads to chronic unresolving pain.

Exposing these sensitized animals to a substance known to cause migraines in humans, such as glyceryl trinitrate, causes the animals to experience a tenfold increase in the sensitivity to light pressure on their foreheads. By sampling cerebral spinal fluid from a major pain center in the base of the rats' brainstems, he was able to show that the increase in pain was causally related to a nearly tenfold increase in glutamate release.

After being introduced to the neurotransmitter modulating potential of noninvasive vagus nerve stimulation (nVNS), Michael tested its effects in his model and showed that administration of nVNS for a brief, two-minute period was able to entirely prevent the increase in pain, along with lowering the rise in glutamate associated with the headache trigger.[67] Even when the nVNS was administered after glutamate levels had risen substantially (approximately halfway to the peak), the therapy was able to turn the glutamate levels around, along with the heightened sensitivity, and return the animal to near normal levels. These data were used as support in the ultimate approval of nVNS as an acute treatment for migraine attacks.

MIGRAINE PREVENTION

Now, inflammation-induced excitotoxicity in the central nervous system, such as what Michael's model generates, and the imbalance of neurotransmitters associated with it, can lead to a susceptibility to various hyperexcitation phenomena. These include seizures and a phenomenon known as cortical spreading depressions (CSDs). CSDs consist of waves of synchronized neural excitation and subsequent inhibition that disable the affected neurons' abilities to function for a period of minutes. CSDs are associated with migraine (and with stroke), and are relatively sporadic. For those who are familiar with migraines, CSDs are believed to be the cause of aura, which is the experience of visual disturbances prior to, or early in, the migraine pain phase. CSDs can affect more than just vision, including disruptions of verbal capability called aphasia.[68]

Research into how migraines work, therefore, includes the study of CSDs. Researchers have identified multiple ways to artificially trigger them in brain tissue.[69] They can be triggered by:

- Placing a small sponge with a high concentration of potassium chloride on the cortex (that locally changes ion gradients);

- Mildly irritating or injuring the tissue (e.g., pricking the surface of the brain with a needle);

- Injecting electrical charge into the tissue (e.g., using a small electrode and applying a current to the tissue);

- Using optogenetic techniques that involve the use of specific frequencies of light to activate the depolarization of neurons genetically altered to be reactive to that frequency; and

- Inducing hypoxia in a region of the brain (which may—or may not—be more relevant for the modeling of ischemic stroke).

If researchers use the injection of charge technique, they can measure the threshold level of charge necessary to initial CSDs. This threshold can be modulated in a variety of ways by certain drugs and neuromodulation therapies. In theory, the lower the threshold, the more likely it is that a CSD will occur, and clinically more likely that a stress of some type will prompt a CSD and migraine. This means that raising the threshold is desirable as a migraine prevention. In this context, an antibiotic called minocycline has the ability to pass through the blood-brain barrier and influence microglial cells to return to their anti-inflammatory state, which raises the thresholds for CSDs.[70]

Richard Kraig of the University of Chicago has published widely regarding the role of microglia in migraine pathogenesis, specifically their effects on CSDs. In a paper published in 2014, he and his colleagues wrote:

> Microglia play an important role in fine-tuning neuronal activity... Excessive synaptic activity is necessary to

initiate spreading depression (SD). Increased microglial production of proinflammatory cytokines promotes initiation of SD, which, when recurrent, may play a role in conversion of episodic to high frequency and chronic migraine.[71]

Cenk Ayata and his colleagues at Harvard Massachusetts General Hospital have spent decades studying CSDs in animal models of both migraine and stroke. In their work, and the work of others, anti-epilepsy drugs, like topiramate, that had been shown to reduce the frequency of migraines, had been shown to reduce CSDs. In fact, the proposed mechanism of action for these drugs was the reduction in hyperexcitability. Unfortunately, it typically takes several weeks to months before these medications reach therapeutically meaningful effectiveness.

In 2012, my close friend and colleague Bruce Simon convinced Cenk to test nVNS as a possible nonpharmaceutical means of raising CSD thresholds. Although he doubted the likelihood of success, Cenk agreed to study the therapy in a simple model of chemically induced CSDs. Over a series of remarkable papers,[72] Cenk and his team demonstrated that nVNS can raise the charge thresholds for electrically triggering CSDs and reduce the frequency of CSDs triggered chemically or optogenetically. Best of all, the benefits that take weeks or months to gain with anti-epilepsy drugs can be attained within a matter of minutes with nVNS.

As a follow-up, Cenk's laboratory has gone on to demonstrate that triggered CSDs have the ability to raise inflammatory cytokine expression (i.e., the relationship between cytokines and CSDs is bidirectional), and that nVNS has the ability to reduce that cytokine expression.

CGRP AND MIGRAINES

This ability to suppress inflammatory cytokines is important in several other aspects of headache pathology, including the release of calcitonin gene-related peptide (CGRP).[73] CGRP is an exceptionally potent vasodilator, which means that it triggers blood vessels to loosen up.[74] It is released by certain neurons in the central nervous system in response to inflammatory cytokine signaling. In this context, the purpose of CGRP release is believed to be its ability to open the blood-brain barrier by causing the cells that form the closely knit barrier to become leaky. This permits the influx of circulating immune cells (monocytes) that infiltrate the brain to become transient proinflammatory macrophages in response to inflammation. CGRP is believed to trigger or at least amplify the development of migraine attacks. Several antibody and small-molecule drugs have been designed to treat headaches by either targeting CGRP directly, or by targeting and blocking the CGRP receptor so the CGRP can't access it.

Paul Durham of the University of Missouri has studied CGRP and migraines for decades, and he has sought safe techniques for inhibiting the effects of CGRP release in the context of headache. Safety of any such agent is important to Paul because he knows that CGRP and its receptors have critical functions throughout the body, for example, in the cardiovascular system and in the retina. It is also crucial for normal wound healing. Thus, in his opinion, CGRP modulation in the central nervous system to prevent migraines must be highly targeted and have minimal off-target effects.[75]

There is, of course, another strategy, which is to inhibit manufacture and release of CGRP only in that setting. As the reader is probably imagining, therapies that suppress or inhibit the inflammatory process might have this desired effect. In 2015, Paul Durham was introduced to the possibility of VNS being just such a targeted therapy and began working with VNS in a groundbreaking model of inflammation-induced migraine susceptibility that he developed.

In several key respects, Paul Durham's animal model of migraine may be as close to the naturally occurring condition as can be generated. In prior models of migraine (or other pain conditions), including those of Michael Oshinsky discussed above, sensitization of a treated animal leaves it with an unnatural chronic pain and correspondingly altered behavior. Subsequent exposure to known migraine triggers causes an amplification of already existing pain responses. That's not the same as having no pain and then experiencing a migraine attack. In Paul Durham's model, he and his colleagues inject a proinflammatory substance, CFA, into the shoulder muscles of rats. In his model, the amount of CFA has been titrated so that it causes a natural inflammatory response that persists for multiple days, but it does not generate a chronic pain state. After eight days of living with the inflammation, however, the animals have become sensitized and are responsive to headache triggers.

In this model, Paul and his team exposed the sensitized animals to a headache trigger called *umbellulone*, and while sensitized animals reliably experienced extreme pain literally causing them to freeze, nVNS was able to prevent that response, whether the nVNS was provided before or after the exposure to the trigger. More interestingly, Durham and his colleagues went on to show that if the animals were given nVNS just twice per day for two minutes each during the initial sensitization phase with the CFA, they never became susceptible to the trigger.

Given the results, Paul went further in his research, testing the animals for evidence of altered cytokine expression. His research, prior to use of nVNS, had demonstrated that sensitized animals exposed to headache triggers showed acute signs of inflammatory cytokine production, and elevated production and release of CGRP. In the studies with nVNS, Paul showed that cytokine production (and the protein expression associated with a proinflammatory response) was suppressed. This was suggestive of a lower level of CGRP production and release.[76]

Intrigued by Paul's findings, Cenk Ayata returned to his own models and studied the effects of CSDs on inflammatory cytokine and CGRP expression, with and without nVNS. According to his published findings, nVNS has the ability to reduce both the expression of inflammatory cytokines triggered by CSDs and the release of CGRP.[77] Given the clinical findings and subsequent FDA clearances for nVNS as a treatment for both acute migraine and as a preventive therapy to reduce the incidence of migraine (and other severe headache conditions), the evidence is strong that nVNS can be a potent therapy against migraine, and that the mechanisms by which it works include glutamate reduction, inhibition of inflammation, and suppression of CGRP expression.

THE VICIOUS CYCLE OF INFLAMMATION

The phenomena that have been discussed in the last few sections involve three central components that form a feedforward loop, or vicious cycle, with each element being exacerbated by the other (see Figure 1).

FEEDBACK LOOP OF NEUROPATHOLOGY

TRAUMA, ISCHEMIA, AND/OR ILLNESS

INFLAMMATION

STRESS, DIET, LACK OF SLEEP, AND/OR TOXINS

Hyperexcitability causes susceptibility to immune triggering events, like CSDs[246]

Cytokines, like TNF-α, alter the expression of neurotransmitters[247]

NEUORONAL HYPEREXCITABILITY

NEUROTRANSMITTER MODULATION

Cytokines and imbalances of neutrotransmitters, like serotonin and glutamate, result in a shift toward a hyperexcitable state[248]

STRUCTURAL ABNORMALITIES AND/OR GENETICS

Figure 1

Inflammation, triggered by an injury or a pathogen, leads to activation of innate immune cells. Within the brain, microglia shift to being proinflammatory and produce cytokines that disrupt the expression of neurotransmitters. This imbalance, which can also arise from stress, diet, and/or toxins, changes the excitation thresholds in the brain, leading to a susceptibility to hyperexcitation phenomena, like CSDs and even seizures.

These events trigger additional inflammation, perpetuating the pathological loop.

VNS has the ability to suppress central (and peripheral) cytokine expression through a reorientation of microglia (and macrophages). The release of acetylcholine from the nucleus basalis of Meynert in the brain (and from ChAT+ cells in the spleen) activate the CAP to return these cells to their homeostatic state.[78] By reducing cytokine expression, levels of inhibitory neurotransmitters, such as serotonin, are increased, and excitatory neurotransmitters associated with the inflammatory response, like glutamate, are moderated. Risks of hyperexcitation phenomena, like seizure and CSDs, are reduced by vagus nerve stimulation because the balance of excitation and inhibition is restored (because imbalances caused by the influence of inflammatory signaling are removed).

VNS impacts the inflammation state, tending to suppress microglial activation and reduce cytokine expression. VNS also activates reuptake mechanisms on astrocytes to take up excessive glutamate, and activates nuclei in the brainstem associated with inhibitory neurotransmitter expression. The suppressive effects on the CNS inflammation state and modulatory impacts on various neurotransmitters' expression levels are likely the general mechanistic rationale(s) explaining the effect of VNS on electrical thresholds and susceptibility to CSDs. VNS also has a suppressive effect on other consequences of hyperexcitation, including, but not limited to, descending inhibition impairment, habituation deficit, central sensitization, and improper pain processing.[79]

STROKE

Stroke is a devastating event that is lethal in up to one-third of cases and typically leaves neurologic deficits in most survivors. Recovery can be grueling, often carrying slim hopes for regaining full function, especially in the elderly. During an ischemic stroke (the vast majority of strokes are of this variety), a region of the brain is deprived of oxygen. Within this region, a population of neurons die from extreme hypoxia. Neurons in a surrounding volume, called the penumbra, are placed under significant oxidative stress.

In this case, oxidative stress refers to a rapid breakdown in OXPHOS (which produces energy ATP) in the mitochondria of the neurons (as well as surrounding cells). To compensate for the lack of ATP generation (without oxygen, aerobic respiration fails rapidly), the desperate cells use a biochemical process called the adenylate kinase reaction to combine two ADP molecules to produce an AMP and an ATP. (Literally taking two molecules that each have two phosphate groups and rearranging them so one has three, and the other has only one.) Cells have a highly sensitive regulating system for maintaining a balance of AMP:ADP:ATP, and this "back-up" pathway to generating ATP produces far more AMP while using up the ADP. This imbalance in AMP:ADP:ATP triggers a cascade of responses all related to AMP-activated protein kinase (AMPK). AMPK can be quite useful in maintaining health and longevity, as we will see in the final chapter, and is being looked at as a target for drug therapies in the context of neuro-ischemic injury. In the case of ischemic stroke, however, extended periods of AMPK activity leads to neuronal cell death.[80]

This ischemia-induced oxidative stress is characterized by a high level of inflammation and CSDs that expand out from the site of the stroke. Recall from the prior section on headache that Cenk Ayata showed CSDs activate microglia, which, in turn, cause the blood-brain barrier to become leaky and allows entry of circulating immune cells. These cells can best be described as being prone to violence. Without protection against the activated microglia and the influx of these additional macrophages, three to five days following an acute stroke, the volume of dead brain tissue (the lesion) can grow by a factor of two or three, even if access to oxygen is restored.

A theory has been proposed that the CSDs are a signal to nerve cells in the surrounding region that oxygen levels may remain low for extended periods, and that the cells should prepare for that new oxygenation state. In fact, CSDs used to precondition brains three days prior to an ischemic event has been shown to reduce the ultimate lesion size by 50 percent.[81] Preconditioning with ischemia has been shown to help reduce transplant rejection resulting from inflammation, and it may involve the activation of the AMPK pathway.

Ilknur and Hakan Ay are a wife and husband research team in the field of stroke. Ilknur is the research scientist, while her husband Hakan is a practicing neurosurgeon, both in the field of stroke. Ilknur's research into the use of VNS for the treatment of stroke has demonstrated the ability of the therapy to reduce the collateral damage (the damage that occurs after the initial hypoxic event) by more than 70 percent.[82]

Analyses of post-stroke brain tissue typically show elevated inflammatory cytokine levels and evidence of damage and death. In the stimulated animals, however, these levels were significantly reduced. Markers of microglial activation were also shown to be reduced.[83]

Ilknur's work was duplicated and extended by Yi Yang at the University of New Mexico in a similar study that also looked at the effects on the blood-brain barrier after the stroke.[84] In the aftermath of a stroke, as stated above, the blood-brain barrier becomes leaky, allowing a free passage for recruited monocytes to enter the brain, exacerbating inflammation. Non-invasive VNS prevented the opening of the barrier, keeping the recruited macrophages out and allowing the lesion to remain close to the original anoxic injury.

These results have led to a clinical study in humans, in which the treatment groups (high and low dosing of nVNS) showed only a 63 percent increase in legion size compared to the 184 percent increase in control groups. Noninvasive VNS appears to have the ability to decrease the collateral damage resulting from inflammation by approximately two-thirds (66 percent) in humans.[85] Much more work needs to be done before nVNS can be approved for the treatment of acute stroke, but intuition suggests (and animal studies have consistently shown) that smaller lesion size will correlate with lower mortality and more rapid recovery of function.

CEREBRAL ANEURYSM

The term *cerebral aneurysm* is often misunderstood. An aneurysm is a bubble-like structure that balloons out from a blood vessel that has weakened and expands at the site of a weakened wall. Although cerebral aneurysms are the under-lying precondition that leads to many hemorrhagic strokes, the aneurysms often form and exist without any symptoms. That's where the good news ends.

Statistics from the Brain Aneurysm Foundation suggest that approximately 1 in 50 adult Americans (6.5 million people) are living with cerebral aneurysms. Further, consider that among these ticking time bombs, one bursts a little more than three times per hour in the US, and half the time, aneurysm rupture is fatal (about one in seven patients don't even make it to the hospital). Half the fatalities are among people aged less than fifty, and close to half a million people in the world die every year of ruptured aneurysms. For those lucky enough to survive, two-thirds are left with permanent neurological deficit. With all of this risk, it is startling and depressing to realize that the spending on cerebral aneurysm research is about two dollars per person afflicted.

One in fifty adults living with cerebral aneurysms does not mean that 2 percent of the population is destined for a grisly hemorrhagic event. Most aneurysms are small, and 50 to 80 percent of all small aneurysms do not rupture. Of course, that still means that at least one in five, and perhaps as many as one in two do rupture! Between 1 and 4 percent of those who arrive at the emergency department for sudden onset severe headaches actually have ruptured aneurysms.

Diagnoses can lead to surgical interventions (like neurovascular coils and clipping procedures) before the rupture, but the location of the aneurysm can prevent surgical access, and as fate would have it, the aneurysms that are most difficult to access are often the ones that are most lethal when they do rupture.

Sufficiently terrified? Well, here is another fact that has public health officials concerned. Hypertension (addressed in the next chapter), which is on the rise, is strongly correlated with the formation of aneurysms. According to the Centers for Disease Control, close to half (47 percent) of adults in America have hypertension, and only one in four have it medically controlled. Majid Ezzati of the School of Public Health at Imperial College in London reported that the number of hypertensive adults in the world doubled during the twenty-nine years from 1990 to 2019.[86]

How do macrophages and microglia play a role in cerebral aneurysm? Recall one of the key roles of microglia during development is to build the vasculature that supplies the brain with blood and oxygen. Within the newly formed blood vessels, the microglia's cousins, vascular and perivascular macrophages, are responsible for remodeling the lining and smooth muscle, which can involve expanding the blood vessel to accommodate high flow, reducing the pressure. One of the steps of this process is to break down the structural links between the cells that line the vessel using matrix metalloproteinases (abbreviated MMPs). When hypertension exists and systemic inflammation is present, these macrophages are triggered to initiate an inappropriate remodeling of the blood vessels, leading to MMP release, weakening the vessel wall.

Given their central role in cytokine expression and MMP release, it is no surprise that the presence of activated macrophages is critical to the aneurysm formation, as well as their progression and ultimate rupture. Given the ability of VNS to quiet inflammatory macrophages, Cenk Ayata also studied its effects in animal models of aneurysm.[87]

More specifically, Cenk and his colleagues tested nVNS to see if it could inhibit the rupture of aneurysms and/or the extent of the damage they cause. In order to generate hypertension, rats underwent unilateral nephrectomies (one kidney was removed) to make them susceptible to medication and salt-induced hypertension. Groups of animals were further separated into mild and severe groups, the difference being in the dosing of the high-salt food and the medication. Rather than injecting MMP, the researchers used a more rapidly acting enzyme called elastase to weaken the cerebral blood vessels. The result of this preparation was multiple aneurysms and spontaneous ruptures (i.e., subarachnoid hemorrhages).

In this study, the nVNS was applied to the active treatment cohorts in each group (moderate and severe) for four minutes per day (two 2-minute doses separated by a five-minute break). This was initiated one day after the elastase was administered and continued until the animals were sacrificed. Among the moderate group, nVNS reduced the aneurysm rupture rate by a remarkable 50 percent (29 percent versus 80 percent). Perhaps as important was the observation that the subarachnoid hemorrhages that did occur were significantly less damaging. In fact, all but one of the VNS-treated animals in the moderate group experienced no neurologic deficits, and the ruptures were all of grade zero (the lowest possible).

Among the severe group (high medication and salt), all animals experienced ruptures by the end of the study. However, the animals in the nVNS group had more than double the survival time, lasting an average of thirteen days before succumbing to an aneurysm rupture versus the animals that did not receive treatment, who survived an average of only six days.

Post-mortem investigations of the animals revealed that the nVNS-treated animals had significantly lower expression of MMP, specifically MMP-9, which led Cenk and his colleagues to conclude, "Noninvasive vagus nerve stimulation has been shown to reduce aneurysm rupture rates and improve outcomes after aneurysm rupture, and may implicate reduced MMP-9 expression as a potential mechanism of action."[88]

Given the role of nVNS in reducing the inflammatory state of macrophages and the critical role inflammatory macrophages play in the creation of cerebral aneurysms, an interesting follow-up study that could be conducted would be to use nVNS during the initial aneurysm-generating phase to see if it can inhibit their creation. Although a human clinical study to demonstrate a lower incidence of aneurysm formation among hypertensive patients would require a very large population and would be confounded by many factors (e.g., adherence to treatment and low-salt diet), the robust safety profile of nVNS along with its relatively low cost make it an easy preventive therapy for those concerned about the risk of developing them.

CHAPTER 4

METABOLIC ACTIVITY AND METABOLIC SYNDROME

At its heart, metabolic activity refers to the generation and utilization of energy in the form of ATP to drive the biochemical reactions that make life work. In the case of a multicellular organism, metabolism can also refer to the movement of energy resources throughout the body, including the creation, storage, transport, and usage of biochemical fuel. Lipids (in the form of fatty acids and triglycerides) and sugars (often in the form of glucose) are the fuel resources most often transported through the body to deliver energy from one place to another. Once they arrive at the target cells in need, these compounds are delivered to the mechanisms (glycolytic enzymes floating throughout the cell, and the mitochondria) that break them down to generate ATP.

Sourcing of these fuels typically comes from the food we eat, either directly from the digestive tract, or later released into the bloodstream by the liver, which has the ability to generate high-energy molecules from stores of fat and a molecule called glycogen. A primary storage site for energy is fat, or adipose cells, and there are several forms of this, typically categorized by color and function (e.g., brown and beige fat, or white adipose tissue).

Metabolic syndrome (or "MetS") is defined by the Mayo Clinic as "a cluster of conditions that occur together, increasing your risk of heart disease, stroke, and type 2 diabetes. These conditions include excess body fat around the waist, high blood sugar, increased blood pressure, and abnormal cholesterol or triglyceride levels."[89]

Data indicates that in most countries of the world, between 12 and 33 percent of adults suffer with MetS. The NIH reports the US at or near the top of that list, with more than one in three adults living with MetS. While the definition of a *pandemic* requires that the disease be infectious, there is no doubt that MetS affects pandemic-like numbers of people.

According to the recommendations of the National Heart, Lung, and Blood Institute and the American Heart Association, a diagnosis of MetS requires three out of the following five observations:[90]

1. Abdominal obesity;
2. Hypertension;
3. Impaired fasting glucose;
4. High triglyceride levels; and
5. Low HDL.

Johns Hopkins School of Medicine's website adds some context to these factors, stating that, "[S]everal factors are interconnected. Obesity plus a sedentary lifestyle contributes to risk factors for metabolic syndrome. These include high cholesterol, insulin resistance, and high blood pressure." In fact, statements to the effect that "abdominal obesity is the most frequently observed component of metabolic syndrome"[91] support the notion that abdominal obesity, itself, may not only be a common risk factor, but in fact may be a direct indication of the root cause; i.e., the other observations required for a diagnosis of MetS are simply consequences of that root cause.

More specifically, a 2015 global survey of obesity reported that over 700 million people (>604 million adults) were obese, and that rates of obesity had doubled over a thirty- to forty-year period in more than a third of countries surveyed, with most other countries also experiencing significant increases.[92] Perhaps more alarming is the fact that the prevalence of MetS is increasing at a rate that mirrors the early to mid-stages, and not the end stages, of a pandemic. Between 1990 and 2015, global rate of death related to high BMI (body mass index) increased by 28.3 percent. The extreme concern being expressed by both healthcare providers and healthcare administrators over MetS is, unfortunately, entirely justified.

These concerns are based on the serious medical risks that follow in the wake of a MetS diagnosis, including stroke, heart attack, limb amputation, liver failure, and recent data suggests significantly elevated risks for neurodegenerative disorders. In fact, a longitudinal study among Finnish men reported that coronary heart disease mortality, cardiovascular disease mortality, and all-cause mortality were 3.77, 3.55, and 2.43 times more likely, respectively, over a twelve-year period for those with MetS.[93]

As discussed in the last chapter, among women who are pregnant, the systemic inflammation associated with MetS increases fetal physical, mental, and emotional developmental problems through in utero programming of microglia and other tissue-resident macrophages. These lead to chronic conditions ranging from respiratory (asthma), neurodevelopmental (autism and schizophrenia), cardiovascular (atherosclerosis) to metabolic (type 2 diabetes) and neurodegenerative (Alzheimer's disease). It is, therefore, not a surprise that identifying the underlying cause of MetS, along with the discovery of new and more effective treatments and/or preventions, are so highly sought after.

As with all organs, macrophages play a critical role in the regulation of fat storage tissue. In fact, it appears that the initial dysfunction that precedes all other MetS symptoms is the failure of adipose tissue-resident macrophages to clear debris (dead cells) when adipose cells are engorged with lipids. This is the efferocytosis function of macrophages that was previously described in chapter 2 with respect to microglia pruning synapses and removing neurons and neural progenitor cells that fail to migrate or differentiate properly.

More specifically, a classic example of healthy efferocytosis by macrophages is the clearance of the hundred billion or so red blood cells (RBCs) that die every single day of our adult lives. As is the case with many cell types, when a fat cell dies (ideally through an organized and preprogrammed process called apoptosis, and not necrosis) an adipose tissue-resident macrophage (ATM) engulfs and removes the dead cell and releases growth factors that promote progenitor cells to create a new adipose cell to take its place. All of this must be carried out in an anti-inflammatory state.

Successful efferocytosis is an efficient and rapid process, but is, in part, rate limited by the size of the cell that is being removed. Adipose tissue cells that are lean at the time they undergo programmed cell death, known as apoptosis, are removed in this efficient manner, despite being near the high end of the size range that healthy ATMs can clear without being coerced into a proinflammatory state. That is, in the case of lean adipose tissue, containing small lipid storage bubbles, clearance by ATMs can remain anti-inflammatory. This stable process goes awry when adipose cells become overly engorged with lipids.

When adipose cells are oversized, the ratio of the volume of tissue to the blood vessels supplying oxygen becomes too large, leading to reduced oxygenation (hypoxia). Hypoxia is a proinflammatory trigger that leads to the recruitment of circulating monocytes into the expanded fat tissue. Influx of recruited circulating monocytes accelerates as fat levels rise, and total macrophage numbers (tissue-resident and newly arrived recruited) increase from approximately 5 to 10 percent in lean individuals to 40 to 50 percent in the white adipose tissue of the morbidly obese.

As the fat cells die and are not cleared or replaced, the lipid contents begin to accumulate in the tissue outside the confines of the cells. That is, there is an increase in extracellular free fatty acid (FFAs) concentrations. Some of the lipids can be engulfed by macrophages, but the excess FFAs in the extracellular matrix have an ability to bind to and activate a set of receptors called toll-like receptors. Toll-like receptors are a group of receptors that have been around for a billion or more years, and they are present in nearly all eukaryotes. Their activation serves a proinflammatory function, reacting to damage or pathogens to shift ATMs into an inflamed state.

Dysregulation of ATMs is further exacerbated as the ATMs that have become proinflammatory, along with recruited macrophages, encircle hypertrophic adipose cells, forming crown-like structures (CLSs), and attempt to clear them. This leads to lipid-bloating of the ATMs, causing them to appear foamy, and ultimately to become dysfunctional and necrotic. Foam cells are characteristic of several related MetS conditions, including atherosclerosis, which is discussed in more detail in a separate section below.

Chronic systemic inflammatory signaling, triggered by the inflamed ATMs and recruited macrophages, induces a number of negative consequences, including insulin resistance, which is described more fully in the section below addressing type 2 diabetes. The term *metabolic syndrome* may apply most directly, however, to the changes in intracellular metabolic activity as mitochondria become markedly dysfunctional in conjunction with elevated levels of inflammatory activity.

INFLAMMATION AND MITOCHONDRIAL DYSFUNCTION

Intercellular inflammatory signaling, such as with circulating cytokines, are designed to alert surrounding (even distant) cells of danger, and to mobilize those cells to defend themselves and the organism as a whole. As described in the context of serotonin synthesis dysregulation, inflammatory cytokines motivate cells to defend themselves, and that defense includes enhanced production of the enzyme indolamine

2,3-dioxygenase (IDO). This reduces serotonin production and enhances kynurenine production. Less serotonin means less melatonin, but an increase in the free radical promoters of the kynurenine pathway, all the way through to quinolinic acid. This loss of serotonin synthesis is the mechanism that explains the results of dozens of studies confirming a positive association between depression and mental and physical fatigue with obesity.[94]

Just as microglia in the brain experienced mitochondrial dysfunction that exacerbated inflammation, ATMs also experience the bidirectional amplification of inflammation and oxidative stress. More specifically, inflammation affects the citric acid cycle (abbreviated TCA), which is at the heart of mitochondrial biochemistry. TCA converts glucose into NADH and FADH to drive the electron transport chain and ATP synthase. In a proinflammatory orientation, ATMs express inducible nitric oxide synthase (iNOS), which, as its name suggests, leads to the synthesis of nitric oxide (NO) and other reactive nitrogen species. These molecules have the ability to disrupt ATP generation. For those who are interested, two important dysregulations of TCA are 1. isocitrate dehydrogenase (IDH) expression, which leads to what's called a continuity failure in TCA (i.e., it stops), and an accumulation of citrate and increased fatty acid synthesis, and 2. decreased activity of succinate dehydrogenase (SDH), which leads to accumulation of succinate (which is proinflammatory) and additional NO production.[95]

Recall that IDO also disrupts melatonin synthesis. Mitochondria generate reactive oxygen species (ROS) as part of their normal function. While antioxidants like superoxide dismutase 1 and 2 are utilized at the mitochondrial membrane to reduce some

ROS, melatonin is a necessary and efficient scavenger utilized by mitochondria to reduce a large fraction of the ROS. Without melatonin, ROS within mitochondria leads to the leakage of free cytochrome-c, which leads to cell suicide. The administration of exogenous melatonin protects against mitochondrial DNA (mtDNA) damage that is caused by ROS*[96] and which can lead to further inflammatory pressure.

These changes within ATMs, especially under prolonged inflammatory conditions, leads to the conversion of these immune cells from being inherently anti-inflammatory into primed cells that react more rapidly and robustly to subsequent proinflammatory signals. These changes that can persist for the rest of a person's life are not yet fully understood; however, it is believed to involve changes in how proteins are expressed within the cell. These changes are referred to generally as *epigenetics*, and involve changes to the DNA and the proteins (histones) around which the DNA is coiled. Histone modifications are known to persist following withdrawal of the initiating inflammatory stimulus and are associated with faster, stronger, and more diversified inflammatory responses to re-stimulation.[97] (How this works is an important topic in the final chapter of this book.) It is important to understand that these epigenetic modifications of nuclear DNA change to the expression of genes that are critical to mitochondrial function for any mitochondria in the cell, and thus permanently disable OXPHOS capability for the cell. This, in part, explains the observed reliance of

---

* Notwithstanding the ability of melatonin to scavenge ROS, melatonin has been shown to mediate reverse electron transport in cancer cells, therein triggering apoptosis and causing cancer cells to commit suicide.

primed macrophages on glycolysis even in the absence of inflammation.

TYPE 2 DIABETES

So, how does all of this inflammation and dysfunction within the ATMs and the enlarged adipose cells affect other systems in the body? The answer lies in the response that many cells, including adipose and muscle cells, have when there is systemic inflammatory signaling present. As cells that are not involved in defense of the body from microbial invasion, they try to avoid being sucked into the maelstrom by producing proteins called suppressors of cytokine signaling (SOCS). These proteins block the upregulation of inflammatory gene expression (through blocking NF-B pathways). In addition to this activity, however, SOCS 1 and SOCS 3 disable the insulin receptor substrate,[98] making these cells, which require insulin signaling for glucose uptake, less sensitive to insulin and thus less able to take in glucose. Remember that the liver is now producing and releasing elevated levels of glucose triggered by this inflammation. Thus, sugar levels in the bloodstream rise (glucose intolerance), as muscle and fat cells are becoming insulin resistant, which is the definition of type 2 diabetes.

As a practical matter, when exposed to high levels of circulating glucose, extracellular proteins become gummed up by this sugar (called glycosylation), which disrupts their function. Among these proteins is hemoglobin. Given the rather well-defined lifespan of a red blood cell (approximately 120 days) the percentage of the hemoglobin molecules that are glycosylated is a reliable measure for how excessive sugar levels have been in the bloodstream over an extended period. This is why hemoglobin A1c (HbA1c)* is used to diagnose and then monitor the health of those with type 2 diabetes. In fact, when glucose levels are high for extended periods, the kidneys are forced to filter it from the blood as a failsafe against toxic levels of glucose, and sugar levels in urine start to rise, which is also a common observation in type 2 diabetes.

In 2011, Wang and colleagues reported on their work suggesting that the cholinergic anti-inflammatory pathway inhibited obesity-induced inflammation and insulin resistance.[99] In fact, mice that have no gene coding for α7-nAChRs (so called 7 knockout animals) produce higher levels of proinflammatory cytokines and become insulin resistant when triggered by excessive free fatty acids. Nicotine, which is an α7-nAChR agonist, suppresses the same free-fatty-acid-triggered inflammation in genetically normal mice, but not the 7KO animals. In fact, nicotine even induced glucose normalization in obese mice significantly, and restored insulin sensitivity. These results and those of others in similar experiments strongly suggested that nVNS might be useful in treating insulin resistance and glucose intolerance.

---

* HbA1c, or A1c, is a measure, typically given as a percentage, of the fraction of hemoglobin protein that has been chemically modified by linking it with a sugar molecule, referred to "glycation." Glycation occurs, to varying degrees, with all circulating proteins, and interferes with their function, which is why high circulating sugar levels is considered unhealthy. Different sugars have different capacities to bind to hemoglobin, with fructose and galactose being relatively strong binders and glucose being a weak binder (which is likely why glucose was selected by evolution to be the sugar of choice for production by the liver).

The study of implanted VNS devices for the treatment of obesity (which has actually received FDA approval) has revealed dramatic reductions in insulin resistance and glucose intolerance.[100] Specifically, this device, the Maestro Rechargeable System (ReShape Lifesciences, Inc., San Clemente, California), which delivers a signal to the vagus nerve just below the diaphragm, demonstrated a reduction in HbA1c of 4 percent after one week, 9 percent after four weeks, 11.5 percent after twelve weeks, and nearly 13 percent at one year. Fasting plasma glucose had an even more precipitous drop of 14 percent at one week, which fell further by 19 percent by twelve weeks and remained at this lower level through one year.

Another implanted device, the TANTALUS™ System (MetaCure Limited, Orangeburg, New York), that stimulates the greater curvature of the stomach, which is highly innervated by the vagus nerve, has been studied in the treatment of type 2 diabetes. In a first study, this therapy delivered a 13 percent drop over a twelve-week period (average HbA1c dropped from 8.4 to 7.3), which fell further to an 18 percent drop by twenty-four weeks. In a follow-up study utilizing the Tantalus-DIAMOND®, data at three years after implantation demonstrated a 14 percent drop in HbA1c within six months and maintained reduction out to thirty-six months.[101]

Noninvasive VNS has also been studied in the treatment of type 2 diabetes. Huang and colleagues published the results of a study using a device that stimulates a tiny branch of a nerve called the tragus that sits in the ear canal and merges into the vagus nerve in the neck. Stimulation of this type is called auricular stimulation (aVNS). It should be noted that the tragus nerve contains only a few hundred nerve fibers, while the vagus contains a thousand times as many fibers. The fibers of tragus also do not project, even after merging in with vagus fibers, directly into the brainstem the way the vagus does. It activates the NTS indirectly through the lateral trigeminal islands.[102] Despite these potential limitations, however, in this study, the treatment group experienced a 24 percent drop in the speed of glucose absorption by cells within two hours at twelve weeks (over baseline), and an 8 percent drop in blood glucose levels after a fast of twelve hours, and maintained this reduction out to twelve weeks.

FATTY LIVER DISEASE

Nonalcoholic fatty liver disease (NAFLD) is a first step on the path toward cirrhosis of the liver caused by a condition known as fibrotic nonalcoholic steatohepatitis (NASH). It is believed to affect nearly 25 percent of the world adult population, with levels approaching 33 percent in many Western countries, and many newly affluent countries in Asia are seeing meteoric rises as well.[103]

The macrophages of the liver are called Kupffer cells, and they represent up to 20 percent of the total number of cells in the liver. As they are located in the liver, they are sensitive to the local activity of liver cells (hepatocytes), such as increased gluconeogenesis. Just like microglia and ATMs (and vascular macrophages we have previously encountered), however, Kupffer cells are also sensitive to autonomic nervous system signaling and systemic inflammatory signals.

To explain, in lean animals, insulin acts locally to cause cells to take up glucose, but also systemically to regulate glucose production. It does this through insulin receptors in the brainstem that then regulate autonomic nervous system signals, including outflow through the vagus nerve. More specifically, modest levels of insulin help to maintain the noninflammatory state among Kupffer cells. This control is actually mediated through activation of the α7-nAChRs on the Kupffer cells. Systemic inflammatory signals associated with obesity induce insulin resistance, which leads the pancreas to increase its release of insulin. These elevated levels of insulin disrupt the vagal control mechanisms, leading to heightened expression of proinflammatory cytokines and chronic hepatic inflammation.[104]

The hepatocytes themselves are also affected by inflammatory signaling and chronic lipid overload in the bloodstream. Failure of fat storage in adipose tissue leads to the accumulation of these fatty acids in the liver. Paradoxically, metabolic studies have revealed that lipogenesis (the manufacture of new lipids) occurs in the liver under these conditions, creating a feed-forward loop.

It turns out that the inflammatory signaling that upregulates lipogenesis leads to intracellular stress at the endoplasmic reticulum. ER stress, as previously mentioned, is coupled with mitochondrial dysfunction through calcium release and cytochrome *c* leakage that can trigger cell death. Of course, hepatocyte apoptosis accelerates activation of Kupffer cells as well as the recruitment of monocytes into the liver, which promotes downstream liver fibrosis.

VNS is in early studies for the prevention and treatment of non-alcoholic steatohepatitis (NASH). In 2017, a team of researchers from Kyoto, Japan, showed that cutting the vagus nerve in animals could accelerate the induction of, and worsen the development of, NASH. Curiously, even the removal of methionine and choline (an important α7-nAChR activator) from the diet could have similar effects and aggravate abnormal lipid metabolism. Subsequent treatment with a chemical bound to α7-nAChRs reduced Kupffer cell inflammation and, in the words of the authors, "contributed to the suppression of NASH progression in its early phase."[105]

In 2018, Li and colleagues, extended these findings, concluding that "activation of α7-nAChR improves energy homeostasis and inhibits inflammation in nonalcoholic fatty liver disease."[106]

A group at Stanford University that I worked with, led by W. Ray Kim, performed a preliminary investigation of liver enzyme levels among patients who had received VNS implants for epilepsy and depression. Among these patients, they identified approximately fifty who had preoperative markers that suggested NAFLD. After the implantations, there was a 33 percent drop in a key enzyme called alanine transaminase, or ALT. ALT is involved in the conversion of protein into energy in the liver, and when it is found in the bloodstream, it is an indication of liver damage. Reductions in ALTs is a sign of reduced metabolic inflammation, lower levels of glucose and lipid synthesis, and less aggregation of fatty acids, all of which are otherwise associated with NAFLD. Translational work remains to be done to determine if noninvasive VNS can provide similar benefits, as it is a much more deployable technology for the volume of individuals currently at risk than a device that requires surgery.

ATHEROSCLEROSIS

Endothelial cells form the inner lining of blood vessels by adhering to one another to form a continuous smooth surface. As we described in the section of chapter 2 focused on cerebral aneurysm, the failure of these cells to remain connected can result in the bubbling out of the vessel wall under pressure spikes, such as are experienced with hypertension. Similar dysfunction of the endothelial cells in arteries and other vessels can be triggered by damage due to hypertension. Coupled with systemic inflammatory signaling and chronically high free fatty acids in circulation, the autonomic nervous system promotes monocyte migration literally into the sidewall of these blood vessels, exacerbating the dysfunction.[107]

More specifically, activation of the sympathetic nervous system facilitates the homing of the monocytes to the site of this damage.[108] These monocytes are programmed to enter into the wall of the blood vessel (called the tunica intima), where they differentiate into recruited macrophages. There, they contribute to the chemical modification of certain lipid molecules (i.e., the oxidation of low-density lipids, LDLs) being transferred across the vessel wall. These oxidized molecules are taken up by these proinflammatory macrophages, leading to their dysregulation of these cells and those around them, including the vascular smooth muscle cells (VSMCs) that form the outside of the vessel wall. Mitochondrial metabolism of fatty acids in these macrophages typically becomes overwhelmed or is inhibited by inflammatory processes, as previously discussed. These macrophages become so filled with lipids, they become foamy looking under a microscope, and are thus referred to as *foam cells*.

In progressing atherosclerosis, which is the formation of lesions within the vessel wall, macrophages and vascular smooth muscle cells (VSMCs) undergo apoptosis.[109] While apoptotic cells are typically cleared quickly when inflammation is minimal or not present, the clearance of these cells is impaired in the diseased blood vessel in much the same way that clearance of enlarged adipose cells is impaired in the adipose tissue.[110]

During normal efferocytosis, macrophages, healthy cells, and apoptotic cells release or express chemical signatures that serve the purposes corresponding to their descriptive names; i.e., "find me," "eat me," and "don't eat me." These signals are exactly analogous, and often literally the same as the molecules that serve the same purposes in the brain! In the inflamed milieu of the growing necrotic core, macrophage/foam cell death stimulates VSMCs to surround them in a last-ditch effort to prevent the inner wall of the vessel from losing integrity. The problem is, these VSMCs have to express "don't eat me" signals to survive, meaning that the clearance of the rest of the necrotic mess is suppressed.[111]

The bursting of these necrotic cores leads to the activation of platelets and the formation of a clot, which can partially or even fully block the flow of blood. These represent high risks for ischemic strokes, heart attacks, and pulmonary emboli (clots that form in the vessels that bring blood to the lungs). Inflammation aggravates all aspects of plaque formation that trigger the thrombotic events.[112]

As described above, the series of pathological events that lead to atherosclerotic plaque formation and elevated risks of clotting events involves the proliferation and recruitment of circulating monocytes. Sympathetic nervous system signaling and chronic inflammation are currently considered as key contributing factors to this process. To the extent that these are features of prolonged hypertrophic adipose tissue (obesity) and insulin resistance (type 2 diabetes), atherosclerosis is regarded as one of the possible symptoms.[113]

As with the prior consequences of obesity, therapies that inhibit inflammation and alter the balance of the autonomic nervous system in the direction of the parasympathetic are of interest in the treatment and/or prevention of atherosclerosis. In the same way that liver tissue was found to have upregulated expression of α7-nAChRs as a way to protect against the ongoing inflammatory cascade, and that absence of these receptors in a knockout animal exacerbated the fatty liver disease, it has been reported that human atherosclerotic necrotic cores and surrounding involved cells express α7-nAChRs, strongly suggesting they are expressed as a defensive move by the tissue to try to reduce inflammation. As the reader will now, no doubt, predict, a series of animal studies have demonstrated that chemical blockers of the cholinergic anti-inflammatory pathway (CAP) result in necrotic core growth and plaque development, while restoration of normal CAP significantly arrested and/or reversed these processes. Similarly, the balance of the current evidence supports the conclusion that α7-nAChR activation inhibits systemic inflammation and alters the inflammatory phenotype of the plaque, consistent with an anti-atherogenic effect.[114]

Is there a role for nVNS in the prevention of atherosclerosis or inhibition of plaque development and/or growth? Multiple lines of reason support that expectation, and several authors have urged that nVNS be studied in this application.[115]

HYPERTENSION

The three major components that control blood pressure maintenance are the heart (the pump), the vasculature (the pipes), and the kidneys (the fluid volume control). The sympathetic nervous system exerts control over all three of these components. In particular, the kidneys regulate blood pressure through the renin-angiotensin-aldosterone system (RAAS), which involves the regulation of salt. This salt is also used to regulate the filtration processes that keep the blood free of toxins. As we have seen previously, inflammation and insulin activate the sympathetic nervous system. Thus, it is no surprise that a large portion of hypertension arises as a consequence of obesity.

Hypertension related to MetS is a form of kidney disease as sodium regulation and blood filtration become dysregulated. Key causative factors of this kidney dysfunction and resulting hypertension include:

- Activation of immune cells and their production of inflammatory cytokines;
- Elevated sympathetic nerve signaling;
- Increased production of angiotensin II and aldosterone; and
- Renal compression by fat in and around the kidneys.

The consequences of obesity on the control of blood pressure by the kidneys arises from a variety of intermediate causes. First, when fat storage function fails, lipids enter circulation and free fatty acids in extracellular spaces activate Toll-like receptors (ancient receptors that recognize damage and/or pathogens), exacerbating local and kidney macrophage activation associated with the onset and progression of hypertension.[116] Second, the physical pressure, caused by lipid accumulation in the kidneys, causes physical damage to the microstructure in the kidneys, leading to a number of physiologic processes becoming dysfunctional, leading to hypertension. Third, of course, insulin resistance and increases in glucose and lipid production from the liver lead to stress on organs, including the kidneys.

Within the kidney, at the microstructural level, elevated insulin and leptin (a key adipokine) levels promote sympathetic signaling and the upregulation of the RAAS. These have been correlated with the development of glomerular hyperfiltration, a state in which the blood flow through the kidneys is significantly increased and has been associated with damage at the level of the individual nephron (the basic filtration unit). This damage leads to a dysregulation in sodium levels, and, of course, activates kidney macrophages, inducing cytokine expression. Renal vasodilatation, a response to inflammatory cytokines, occurs to restore sodium balance; however, this exacerbates glomerular hyperfiltration. This creates a feed-forward loop, making hypertension a progressive disorder.[117]

An additional component of hypertension is mitochondrial dysfunction. Mechanical shearing forces and pressure upregulate an enzyme called NADPH oxidase expression, which leads to the increased production of damaging molecules (e.g., ROS) that damage mitochondria. In turn, mitochondrial dysfunction leads to a shift from aerobic respiration (lots of ATP per glucose molecule) to anaerobic respiration (glycolysis, and inefficient ATP production), and correspondingly reduced oxygen demand.

Endothelial cells are sensitive to changes in oxygen levels in circulation, leading to vasoconstriction as a consequence of relative hypoxia.[118] This vasoconstriction leads to higher blood pressure (same volume, less space).

VNS leads to the release of acetylcholine and the activation of the CAP, which reduces systemic inflammation, preserves mitochondrial function, and reorients macrophages to their homeostatic and anti-inflammatory state. As described above, all of these effects should provide benefit in preventing the onset of and/or treatment of hypertension. Animal studies of induced hypertension in salt sensitive rats demonstrated that a four-week cycle of VNS treatments significantly reduced mean arterial pressure compared with sham treated rats.[119]

Human studies of VNS in the treatment of obesity and type 2 diabetes, previously cited, also reported reductions in blood pressure among those with hypertension. Specifically, a study of the implanted Tantalus device showed that among the forty-four of fifty patients who entered the study with an average blood pressure reading of 144/89 mmHg dropped to 131/80 mmHg.[120] Similarly, a study of an implanted VNS device for the treatment of obesity demonstrated that among the hypertensive subgroup of participants, the average blood pressure readings dropped from 140/88 mmHg to 130/78 mmHg within one week and maintained that reduction at four, twelve, and twenty-six weeks, and averaged 128/78 mmHg at one year post initiation of VNS therapy.[121]

ALZHEIMER'S DISEASE AS TYPE 3 DIABETES

Alzheimer's disease (AD) is a devastating chronic neurodegenerative disorder characterized by dementia. When studied at the microscopic level, AD is associated with a number of observations, including:

- The formation of plaque-like lesions between neurons comprised of a protein called *amyloid* (amyloid aggregates);
- Structural damage within neurons related to the deposition of an activated protein called *tau* (neurofibrillary tangles);
- Inheritance of the gene for apolipoprotein E4 (genetic predisposition);
- Oxidative stress (mitochondrial dysfunction);
- Neuronal death; and
- A general atrophying of the central nervous system.

Ticking down this list, the presence of high levels of amyloid beta and phosphorylated tau have led to significant resources being spent targeting these proteins in the hopes of treating or delaying the onset of the clinical symptoms, such as the inability to form new memories and progressive dementia.[122] Unfortunately, there has been little success and much failure of these approaches.

Studies of the functions of apolipoprotein E have revealed that the protein has critical activities in the brain, one of which is related to lipid transport among cells throughout the CNS. Further, it has been shown that this E4 variant is dysfunctional with respect to this function. More specifically, one of the leaders in the study of apolipoprotein E, Robert Mahley, stated:

> In multiple pathways affecting neuropathology, including Alzheimer's disease, apoE acts directly or in concert with age, head injury, oxidative stress, ischemia, inflammation, and excess amyloid peptide production to cause neurological disorders, accelerating progression, altering prognosis, or lowering age of onset. We envision that unique structural features of apoE4 are responsible for apoE4-associated neuropathology.[123]

This is an important clue into how metabolic dysfunction secondary to obesity and lipid dysregulation might lead to and/or exacerbate AD. Before we go into the role of MetS in AD, it is important to see how the remaining observations might relate to this perspective.

Previous discussion has covered that mitochondrial and immune (microglial) dysfunctions are associated with chronic inflammation. Mitochondria in microglia of patients with AD typically exhibit a dysfunctional state, and microglia in these patients exhibit an inappropriate orientation toward aggressive synaptic pruning; that is to say, a dysregulated homeostatic function that dismantles the connectivity of the brain.[124]

So, how do mitochondrial dysfunction, microglial activation, and lipid dysregulation, all of which are aspects of MetS, relate to AD? In 2005, Sandra de la Monte and colleagues published a paper first referring to AD as type 3 diabetes. Specifically, the authors cite "accumulating evidence that reduced glucose utilization and deficient energy metabolism occur early in the course of [Alzheimer's] disease, suggests a role for impaired insulin signaling in the pathogenesis of AD."[125]

In support of this, a 2008 paper reported on a remarkable Swedish longitudinal study that followed 2,269 men for thirty-two years. It revealed that low insulin production due to chronic status as type 2 diabetics at age fifty was shown to impart a 50 percent greater risk for developing AD when compared with those having normal insulin levels.[126] Interestingly, this association was higher among patients who did *not* have the genetic predisposition to AD associated apolipoprotein E4. This suggests that the enhanced risk associated with metabolic dysregulation that comes from chronic diabetes and the loss of insulin production is already factored in by the presence of apolipoprotein E4. Just to make sure that point is fully appreciated, the fact that insulin dysregulation leads to a stronger elevation in AD risk among people without the apolipoprotein E4 variant, but E4 itself elevates the risk of AD, strongly suggests that they are working along the same pathways (e.g., lipid dysregulation). Think about it this way—if the police place a boot on your car, it will likely reduce the number of miles that the car can be driven, but it won't have that effect if the car engine is broken already.

Wait for it ... subsequent work has shown that insulin dysregulation is a causative factor in the phosphorylation of tau protein, the formation of neurofibrillary tangles, and the formation amyloid plaques. So, the three theories of AD pathogenesis can actually be knit together in a meta-theory based on chronic inflammation and the lipid dysregulation and metabolic dysfunction that comes from obesity. First, systemic inflammation associated with obesity leads to insulin dysregulation, which is tied to phosphorylation of tau protein and plaque formation. Similarly, inflammatory cytokines disrupt mitochondrial function, which leads to damage and the possibility of cell suicide. Finally, the microglia that are activated begin to aggressively misapply their synaptic pruning function.[127]

As we have discussed, VNS has the capacity to similarly shift the posture of macrophages and microglia, and reduce cytokine expression. Clinical studies of VNS in the treatment of AD are limited, but one trial conducted in Sweden demonstrated promising results. In a first follow-up at three months after initiation of treatment among AD patients, 70 percent of patients experienced at least a 3-point improvement on the Alzheimer's Disease Assessment Scale—cognitive subscale (ADAS-cog), and 90 percent experienced at least a 1.5-point improvement on the Mini-Mental State Exam (MMSE). A subsequent follow-up at one year showed that these numbers had slipped to 41 percent and 71 percent, respectively, but still, 71 percent improved or remained stable on the Clinician Interview-Based Impression of Change (CIBIC+).[128] A criticism of this first study is that the patients being treated were already diagnosed with moderate to severe AD, and were likely too far gone to be sufficiently helped. Current studies are underway with noninvasive VNS in mild AD, with readouts scheduled over the next several years. With the safety of nVNS, it would be possible to study patients who are only experiencing mild cognitive impairment (MCI) to see if the progression can be entirely prevented.

CHAPTER 5

....

WOMEN'S REPRODUCTIVE HEALTH

During gestation, the groundwork for future reproduction is already being built. For males, the testes prepare to produce sperm, and for females, the ovaries, fallopian tubes, and uterus develop. In both sexes, the first stage of breast tissue development occurs. Later, during puberty, this tissue is dismantled in males. Conversely, during puberty, females experience the second stage of breast development involving the construction of milk ducts and other tissue to support lactation. The third stage of breast development occurs for females during pregnancy, with the development of fully functioning lactating tissue. This tissue is partially dismantled again after the cessation of breastfeeding.

All of these organs are constructed by, or under the direct signaling control of, tissue-resident macrophages. The maintenance, remodeling (during sexual maturation, through pregnancy, and during menopause), and support of these organs is also the responsibility of these macrophages. As will be discussed in the following sections, dysfunctional and/or symptomatic experiences associated with reproductive tissue nearly always involve, and are very often driven by, the activation of these macrophages into an inflammatory state. In this state, as we have seen in the brain and in the multiple systems associated with metabolic syndrome, macrophages disengage from the maintenance, remodeling, and support of the organs, leading to dysregulation and dysfunction.

From the time of puberty onward, the female immune and autonomic nervous systems function in harmony to enable fertility. In 1980, Espey formulated the hypothesis that ovulation is driven by inflammatory pathways. That is not to imply that healthy fertility is an inflammatory event; it just shares a lot of common pathways. More specifically, ovulation is triggered by a surge of luteinizing hormone that leads to the expression of signaling molecules and metabolic pathways also associated with inflammation. Tissue-resident macrophages are activated as they moderate extensive alterations of follicular structures, including extensive extracellular matrix remodeling and rapid angiogenesis, which ultimately leads to follicular rupture and oocyte release.[129] This process involves inflammatory signaling, but also requires anti-inflammatory signaling in order for the female to carry a fetus to term. This is similar to how debris clearance, called efferocytosis, which is anti-inflammatory, mimics the inflammatory phagocytosis of pathogens.

In coordinating all aspects of ovulation, these tissue-resident macrophages remain responsive to autonomic signaling, ensuring the release of a mature egg cell, the traversal of the egg through the fallopian tubes, potential conception, and either implantation and growth of the embryo within the uterus, or the ejection of the egg and the lining of the uterus that had been prepared for implantation of a fertilized egg.

In the case of pregnancy, both maternal and placental macrophages and the autonomic nervous system of the mother (initially) and fetus (during the latter stages of gestation) work together to:

- Construct and maintain the temporary organ that is the combined uterus and placenta;
- Ensure proper gestation and monitoring of the developing fetus, ensuring all aspects of growth are sustained or, in the event of genetic or congenital defects, the natural termination of the pregnancy;
- Produce fully functioning lactating tissue;
- Initiate labor;
- Initiate lactation;
- Return the uterus to its pre-pregnancy state;
- Restore the menstrual cycle;
- Dismantle the lactating tissue when nursing is discontinued; and
- Discontinue fertility at menopause.

With every change outlined above, some of which will be described in greater detail in the following sections, dysregulation of the immune system and/or autonomic nervous system can cause symptoms ranging from premenstrual pain, mood dysregulation, and digestive issues, to gestational conditions, such as gestational diabetes and preeclampsia. Infertility (POF), endometriosis, polycystic ovarian syndrome (PCOS), and the various menopausal symptoms of body-temperature regulation, and other uncomfortable vasomotor experiences, are related to autonomic and immune challenges, as well.

Given that VNS has been shown to increase parasympathetic activity and reduce inflammation levels, and more particularly shift macrophages away from a proinflammatory posture to the homeostatic focus, it is not surprising that it supports healthy reproductive function.

For example, early in pregnancy, an elevation in vagal tone is normal.[130] Unpleasant and even dangerous pregnancy symptoms from nausea to gestational diabetes are associated with a failure of vagal tone to rise. Later in life, vasomotor symptoms of menopause can be reduced by vagus nerve activation.

OVULATION AND MENSTRUATION

Up to 80 percent of women experience some form of premenstrual symptom(s), including symptoms of fatigue, irritability, mood swings, depression, abdominal bloating, breast tenderness, acne, changes in appetite, and food cravings, collectively referred to as premenstrual syndrome (PMS), with some studies suggesting that more than half of these women seek out medical advice for their management.[131] While much emphasis has been placed on the roles of estradiol and progesterone released after ovulation, a reduced availability of serotonin seems to be involved, with some research implicating the role of inflammatory cytokines in affecting brain neurotransmitter expression. The severe form of PMS, called premenstrual dysphoric disorder, is often treated with selective serotonin reuptake inhibitors—a medication designed to alter synaptic serotonin levels when serotonin levels are believed to be abnormally low and a cause of symptoms.[132]

As previously described, serotonin has multiple roles in health, in the central nervous system (e.g., mood, sleep, and pain regulation through descending inhibition) and with respect to metabolic function, specifically with respect to efficient oxidative phosphorylation within mitochondria (e.g., as a precursor for the critical antioxidant, melatonin). Serotonin also plays an important role in digestion (e.g., motivating peristaltic motion). As discussed, inflammatory cytokines negatively affect serotonin in multiple ways. First, through the upregulation of indolamine 2,3 dioxygenase, tryptophan metabolism is shifted away from serotonin synthesis. Second, serotonin transporters (SERT), which are the reuptake mechanisms targeted by SSRI and SNRI drugs, are upregulated by inflammatory cytokines.[133]

The menstrual cycle involves a rise in sympathetic activity and inflammatory cytokine production that typically peaks right before menstruation. Following menses, there is a steady decline in circulating cytokines throughout the follicular phase. As stated previously, a surge of luteinizing hormone (LH) released by the pituitary gland triggers the beginning of ovulation. This bolus of LH activates a mild, but clearly measurable, expression of inflammatory cytokines and chemokines that actually attract monocytes (that differentiate into recruited macrophages) that engage with preovulatory follicles. These recruited macrophages, which are proinflammatory by nature, amplify the local proinflammatory cytokines necessary to stimulate ovulation and promote oocyte maturation. In support of this is the fact that dual treatment with the inflammatory cytokine, TNF-α, along with LH, significantly increases the ovulation rate, while blocking TNF-α inhibits ovulation.[134]

A cross-sectional study across a racially/ethnically diverse group of women (n = 2939) demonstrated a significantly positive association between high-sensitivity C-reactive protein (hs-CRP) level >3mg/L and premenstrual mood symptoms, abdominal cramps/back pain, appetite cravings/weight gain/bloating, and breast pain.[135]

In parallel with the inflammatory fluctuations, there is a shift in autonomic nervous system activity throughout the menstrual cycle. The luteal phase is associated with an elevated level of sympathetic activation. This appears to be correlated with progesterone levels, and there is a strong indication that increased sympathetic activity during the late luteal phase might be the cause of premenstrual syndrome (PMS) in some women.[136]

Autonomic nervous system activity is tightly associated with inflammation; as one author expressed it, "A major purpose of increased SNS (sympathetic) activity is nourishment of a continuously activated immune system at a systemic level." Altered functioning of the ANS in the late luteal phase also corresponds with premenstrual symptoms, and studies indicate that when symptoms become more severe (as seen in women with PMDD), vagal tone is more depressed than normal.[137]

Vagus nerve stimulation is a direct way to influence the ANS, increasing the parasympathetic tone and reducing the effects of sympathetic activation, including excessive inflammation.

PREGNANCY AND INFERTILITY

The most common cause of female infertility is premature ovulatory failure, or POF, the primary cause of which is inflammation. Heart rate variability (HRV) has been shown to be lower among patients with POF,[*138] suggesting a role for autonomic nervous system dysfunction and vagal insufficiency in the condition.

Tissue remodeling is a macrophage function that necessitates precise coordination, and in the case of ovulation and maintaining female fertility, macrophage distraction by inflammation or excessive sympathetic signaling can disrupt the process. This means that significant stress can disrupt the exquisitely timed flow of events that are critical for ovulation to occur, and the monthly cycle literally fails to produce a viable egg. The most widely known form of this dysfunction is the one that occurs among women suffering with eating disorders, like anorexia, who cease having a regular cycle because their bodies are under a chronic state of malnutrition. This same phenomenon can occur on the opposite end of the physiological spectrum among women who overtrain for athletic competitions and are under chronic physical stress.[139]

VNS has been shown to positively affect stress response, reducing sympathetic activation, and reducing inflammation. In 2011, Huang and colleagues published a survey of the studies using acupuncture techniques to activate the auricular tragus nerve that enhanced pregnancy rates.[140]

---

* Heart rate variability is a measure of the beat-to-beat difference in the rate that the heart is beating. Given the dual control of the sympathetic nervous system trying to accelerate the heart, and the parasympathetic influence which slows the heart, a high degree of variability is considered a sign of health and a strong parasympathetic tone.

Similarly, in 2019, Kusuma and colleagues published results in IVF patients demonstrating that acupuncture that included auricular stimulation produced statistically significantly more mature oocytes and resulted in a greater percentage of successful pregnancies.[141] Anecdotal reports from multiple nVNS users support the possibility that certain challenges getting pregnant can be resolved with regular use of the therapy.

Polycystic ovarian syndrome (PCOS) is another reproductive system condition, characterized by symptoms ranging from pain and altered ovarian morphology to infertility. Interestingly, it has been classified as a metabolic condition, given the role that insulin dysregulation plays in the condition. The potential use of VNS in the treatment of PCOS has recently gained attention with the publishing of a 2023 paper by Zhang and colleagues out of China. In this paper, the authors assert that VNS should be studied as a treatment for PCOS, because "[a]bnormalities in the ANS play an important role in the progression of ovarian pathological conditions, such as PCOS."[142] Clinical studies using VNS to treat PCOS have not yet commenced, but Zhang, et al. have laid out a viable rationale for its efficacy.

MENOPAUSAL SYMPTOMS

Activity in the autonomic nervous system and among tissue-resident macrophages both respond to, and influence, the expression of hormonal changes during menopause. Symptoms that are commonly experienced during menopause that result from these changes include mood dysregulation, fatigue, and hot flashes during the day and night sweats during sleep. "Hot flashes [are] the most common menopause-related complaint of peri- and post-menopausal women in Western countries."[143]

According to research, changes in the balance between sympathetic and parasympathetic activity is due to estrogen withdrawal. Not surprisingly, ANS dysregulation (and inflammation) are key underlying causes of many symptoms of menopause. This has been demonstrated by several lines of study, beginning with the fact that yohimbine, a compound that increases central sympathetic activation, provokes hot flashes, and clonidine, a drug that reduces sympathetic activation, ameliorates them. Multiple studies have shown HRV is significantly decreased during daily hot flashes relative to periods preceding and following. Similarly, moderate to severe hot flashes and sleep problems are related to an increase of sympathetic nerve activity and a decrease in parasympathetic tone. For example, in a study conducted among women suffering night sweats, a measure of autonomic nervous system activity showed "a decrease in vagal [parasympathetic] activity, at the onset of a hot flash compared to baseline and pre-flash [and] ... the magnitude of the hot flash, i.e., skin conductance amplitude, was associated with increased heart rate and decreased vagal tone."[144]

This increased sympathetic activation drives inflammation. Unsurprisingly, in a study of cytokine expression in more than 200 women, stratified by frequency and severity of hot flashes, a positive correlation between severity and cytokine level was seen. Measurements of nine circulating cytokines/chemokines demonstrated that the more severe the symptoms, the higher the levels of TNF-α, IL-6, IL-8, and MIP1β. These data are consistent with prior data associating hot flashes with inflammatory cytokines, even in otherwise healthy postmenopausal women.[145]

As we have discussed, parasympathetic activity is often suppressed by enhanced sympathetic activity, and vice versa. Most importantly, inflammation is suppressed by parasympathetic activation. Thus, if enhanced sympathetic activity triggers or exacerbates hot flash symptoms, parasympathetic activation (VNS) should be an effective suppressor of hot flashes.

In fact, activation of the parasympathetic through natural means (i.e., exercise, deep breathing, ice baths, and meditation) have been shown to reduce hot flashes and elevate perimenopausal mood. Observational studies have associated high levels of exercise with a lower hot flash frequency and shown that, conversely, lack of physical exercise can increase their frequency. A 2016 study tested the hypothesis directly and found that a sixteen-week exercise training intervention significantly reduced hot flash weekly frequency by approximately 62 percent. As of 2023, while official statements by the North American Menopause Society position the non-hormone management of vasomotor symptoms isn't dispositive, the majority of evidence from randomized control trials indicate that aerobic and resistance exercise training lead to a decrease in subjectively experienced hot flashes.[146]

Although evidence regarding meditation and hot flashes is conflicting, a study of meditation on hot flashes was published in 2020 by Sung and colleagues in Korea. Sixty-five healthy women included thirty-three meditation practitioners and thirty-two non-meditation controls. The meditation group showed a trend of reductions in depression and irritability.[147]

Similarly, another natural technique for activating para-sympathetic tone, deep breathing, has been studied for its effectiveness in reducing hot flash burden among menopausal women. A 2019 study enrolled eighty women having experienced abrupt surgical menopause into two groups: forty women who practiced deep breathing multiple times per day for three weeks, and a control group of forty women who did not. Statistically significant differences in hot flash frequency was evident between the groups by the second week and continued to improve in the third week. Additionally, the quality of daily life activities was also significantly improved by week three.[148]

VNS enhances parasympathetic activity, decreases sympathetic tone, and inhibits inflammation. It is, therefore, not surprising that evidence has begun to accumulate that VNS reduces the burden of hot flashes. Interestingly, hot flashes are often experienced by men with prostate cancer who undergo certain chemotherapeutic therapies (similar to the hormonal withdrawal experienced by women in menopause). In a study of tragus nerve stimulation with acupuncture among a small pilot population, an excellent reduction of hot flash symptoms, along with improved quality of life and sleep, was observed.[149]

Regarding the potential of VNS to elevate mood otherwise impacted by menopause, we have already described the mechanisms (serotonin expression and reduction in inflammation) of VNS in depression, and the fact that it was already approved by the FDA for the treatment of medically refractory depression based on numerous studies. Studies in the treatment of various anxiety conditions have also demonstrated benefits.[150]

Sleep disruption and fatigue are also common symptoms of menopause. Not surprisingly, sleep disruption is associated with increased activity of the sympathetic nervous system[151] and inflammation.[152] Short-term consequences of sleep disruption include decreased stress resilience, lower mood, reduced pain tolerance and enhanced pain perception, as well as cognitive, memory, and learning deficits. VNS has been shown to improve the restorative quality of sleep and expand the duration of deep sleep.[153]

It is worth noting that implanted VNS, which are typically pro-grammed to deliver stimulation once every five minutes day and night, have shown a small but identifiable increase in mild apnea risk. There is evidence that this risk is related to the implantation technique, and it has not been observed among users of noninvasive technologies.[154] Even if there were any transient effect of the VNS therapy itself on sleep apnea, and none has been identified, because noninvasive technologies are not used during sleep, and they are typically used far less frequently than implanted devices, it is unlikely that apnea will emerge as a risk for nVNS.

Given everything previously explained about inflammation and mitochondrial function, is it any wonder that fatigue is a common complaint among women going through menopause? Noninvasive VNS has been studied in cohorts of primary Sjogren's Syndrome patients (an autoimmune condition that impacts fluid production glands, impacting salivary, mucus, and tear production). In this study, forty participants with PSS were randomly assigned to use active or sham nVNS devices twice daily for fifty-four days. Multiple patient-reported mea-sures of fatigue were collected prior to initiating a fifty-six-day trial as well as at the end of the study. Neurocognitive tests and inflammatory markers were also compared between active and sham throughout the study. Fatigue scores were significantly reduced by the end of the study in the nVNS group only. There were also significant improvements in the neurocognitive testing (the areas of the brain associated with creativity and thought improved as the fatigue scores went down).[155]

POST-MENOPAUSAL RISKS

The uncomfortable symptoms of menopause, including fatigue, depression, hot flashes, and sleep troubles turn out to be far more than just an inconvenience, but rather are harbingers of future medical problems that can be far more serious. The timing and severity of these symptoms, called vasomotor symptoms, have been correlated with higher risks of several serious medical conditions during the post-menopausal period. Early and infrequent symptoms are associated with fewer complications, while late and frequent/severe vasomotor symptoms are associated with conditions, including cardiovascular disease, atherosclerosis, stroke, metabolic disease, osteoporosis, depression, and memory problems.[156] Of course, all have been shown to be related to heightened sympathetic nervous system activity and inflammation. (The one of the above conditions that has not been previously covered is osteoporosis, which has been related to altered macrophage activity; in this case, the macrophages of bone, which are called osteoclasts.)

Bone formation in gestation, growth during childhood, and remodeling in response to stresses throughout life are all managed by the tissue-resident macrophages of the skeletal system, osteoclasts. These cells are most well-known for their ability to dismantle bone matrix, but it is their response to normal wear and tear that leads to the anti-inflammatory process that triggers the resorption of worn bone material that is not functioning and the promotion of their partner cells, the osteoblasts, to remodel and replace the bone that is not functional. This is reminiscent of the previously described macrophage function of efferocytosis (the noninflammatory debris clearance function used in adipose tissue turnover, blood vessel formation, neural development, and synaptic pruning).

In fact, the parallel between the remodeling of bone and blood vessel growth and remodeling is uncanny. In the development of a network of blood vessels, the macrophages coordinate the growth of a seemingly random connected tangle of vessels that is then sculpted back to an efficient network that maintains smooth blood flow with sufficient oxygen carrying capacity to handle the demands of the tissue it supplies. The initial deposition of bone matrix, for example in the case of a broken bone, is in the form of a thick callous, which is then optimized through a slow removal of bone matrix and mineralization that is superfluous. Just as aspects of autism spectrum disorder or Alzheimer's disease can be considered a microgliosis (a disease caused by microglial dysfunction), and peripheral vascular disease can be observed to be a failure of the perivascular and vascular macrophages to maintain the micro vessel structures, osteoporosis can be considered a dysfunctional remodeling process by osteoclasts.

Not surprisingly, the peak of vasomotor symptoms, which includes hot flashes, coincides with the peak acceleration in bone loss. Long-term studies over the decade of menopause and post-menopause have found that women with moderate to severe vasomotor symptoms experienced greater demineralization (lower bone mineral density as measured in the spine and at the head of the femur) and increased rates of hip fractures compared with women who have minimal to no vasomotor symptoms. Again, during menopause, reduced hormone levels are linked to increases in the expression of cytokines that stimulate osteoclast and osteoblast formation, leading to increased bone turnover and eventually bone loss.[157]

The ability of VNS to modulate inflammation and autonomic nervous system activation strongly suggests that it can be beneficial in preventing bone loss during and after menopause. Ma and colleagues found that activation of the cholinergic anti-inflammatory pathway through activation of α7-nAChRs reduced bone demineralization in an animal model of bone loss. In their words:

> [I]nflammatory factors are involved in osteoporosis pathogenesis. After 6 or 12 weeks [on an α7-nAChR agonist], [bone density [was] ... remarkably potentiated in the drug treatment group ... Agonists of α7-nAChR can up-regulate estrogen receptor expression and may prevent the occurrence and development of osteoporosis.[158]

Switching gears, as discussed previously, it is not simply hot flashes that correlate with the development of more serious medical problems. The experience of hot flashes coincides with greater self-reported anxiety and depressive symptoms, and that too is associated with chronic inflammation. Thus, if menopause is marked by an increased prevalence of mood symptoms in midlife women, including anxiety and depression, concerns have been raised that increased mood symptoms in midlife alone may be associated with an increased risk of other adverse health outcomes.[159]

More specifically, prior research in men and non-menopausal women has suggested that both anxiety and depression may be associated with alterations in cardiac autonomic function, particularly parasympathetic dysfunction (low vagal tone) as measured by heart rate variability (HRV). Increased sympathetic and decreased parasympathetic activation have in turn been associated with adverse cardiovascular outcomes and mortality in patients with cardiovascular disease, such as coronary artery disease and chronic heart failure, as well as higher rates of chronic diseases that increase incidence of cardiovascular disease, such as obesity, diabetes, and hypertension.[160]

Researchers have found that mood and anxiety symptoms during menopause were similarly associated with lower levels of resting cardiac parasympathetic activity, and greater levels of anxiety were associated with higher levels of cardiac sympathetic activity. These data raise concerns, as women with increased anxiety and depressive symptoms likely have an elevated risk of future cardiovascular issues, ranging from hypertension and atherosclerosis to heart attacks and strokes.[161]

The number of different medical conditions that arise during and after menopause among women who experience autonomic dysregulation and inflammation raises the question as to whether other comorbid states driven by this sort of sympathetic overactivity exist. In the next chapter we will see that this is certainly the case, and it may explain one of the most expensive aspects of healthcare.

CHAPTER 6

MULTISYMPTOM SUFFERERS

I previously mentioned that my father was an OB-GYN. When I was old enough to recognize the hours that OBs kept, being at the mercy of when his patients went into labor, even if it was at two-thirty in the morning in the middle of January, I asked why he chose that field of medicine. He had a curious answer. He said he liked OB because the Monday morning conversations among the doctors who dealt with cancer, heart disease, or other problems were often centered around who had died over the weekend. Among the OBs, however, the conversation was about who had had a child and what new person had been born. To him, OB just seemed bright and optimistic, while the other fields were heavier and often fatalistic.

Despite the fact that the field holds a lot optimism, my father still encountered many patients whose medical problems just seemed to deteriorate despite everything he tried. I don't mean that they were dying, but rather that their quality of life was plummeting. These patients had started out as healthy and vibrant young women, and yet as they moved into their thirties and forties, their health devolved. They had migraines, complained of depression or anxiety, and suffered with allergies, sinus problems, and even a late onset of asthma. Some reported uncomfortable gastric motility problems, like IBS or reflux, and many were dealing with issues getting to sleep or staying asleep. In other cases, the women were experiencing all-over pain or debilitating fatigue. These problems can affect men, too, but across the board, these symptoms seem to affect women far more than men. For example, migraine affects three times as many women as men, and close to 90 percent of patients with fibromyalgia are women.

Many of my father's colleagues recognized the same pattern among their patients, but they would quickly become frustrated by their inability to effectively treat them. Many chalked the women's problems up to "female hysterics" and referred to them as "crazy." (Ugly medical history fact: the term *hysterectomy* actually comes from the 19th century belief that performing this surgery removed the hysteria from women!) Others claimed that women lied, sometimes even saying it to their faces. Fortunately, my father was intellectually honest enough to admit that the patients were sane and honest. He was also humble enough to accept that, despite his Georgetown Medical School degree, he just didn't know how to treat them.

Fast-forwarding twenty-five years, I found myself as the founder and CEO of a company developing a noninvasive vagus nerve stimulation device to treat headache conditions. At the time, I had become fascinated by the ability of the therapy to address an eclectic mixture of conditions, ranging from epilepsy and depression, to obesity, migraine (of course), asthma, and even rheumatoid arthritis. A study with promising effects in fibromyalgia was the straw that broke the camel's back for me. The potential for this therapy to help so many people was overwhelming, but I needed to understand the limits of what we were dealing with.

Keeping in mind that the original product was FDA cleared for treating headaches, I found an article from 2004, written by two nurses, Jacqueline Pesa and Maureen Lage. They had been interested in how the costs of managing mental health (depression and anxiety) patients changed if patients also suffered with migraines. Their results showed that the comorbidity of migraine and mental health condition made patients far more expensive than patients with only one condition. Since VNS could arguably treat both the mental health conditions and the headaches at the same time, I suspected that meant the economic benefits would be quite significant if these patients who were so expensive simply started using VNS. If I could show that, it would be a powerful argument in favor of paying for the therapy. It was around that time that I became aware of the work by Dr. Muhammad Yunus on the comorbidity that suggested a phenomenon called *central sensitization* might be underlying the problem.[162]

CENTRAL SENSITIZATION

To understand central sensitization, imagine seeing a close friend with a severe scowl on his or her face. Your brain immediately recognizes the expression and creates an expectation for your friend to engage with you as he or she does when in a bad mood. This is where it gets interesting, because your brain is now making a prediction regarding the character of the input that it has yet to receive. Neuroscientist Anil Seth describes the brain as a "prediction machine."[163] What does he mean? He means that when your friend actually starts speaking, you are liable to interpret what he or she is saying as a complaint, or as an expression of frustration, or even as outright anger. That is, the expectations you have create a cognitive and emotional framework through which you will interpret all inputs from your friend. The brain uses prior perceptions of information it received in the past, which are, in and of themselves subject to prior interpretations, to predict the meaning of currently received inputs. If that seems hard to comprehend, think again about your friend with the scowl on his or her face and ask yourself how you would respond if asked, "And how's your day going?" Would you reply with a smile and say, "Great, how're you doing?" or would you say with concern, "I'm all right, but is everything OK with you?"

Now, imagine that same prediction machine interpreting the input of pressure against your arm. The brain has to interpret whether the input coming through the nerve endings in your skin is a threat, in which case a pain response is appropriate in order to motivate you to move away from the pressure, or if it is benign, your brain will consciously perceive the pressure for a moment and then mute that input, allowing it to recede into the background. When I am speaking with an audience of people on this topic, I often ask them to raise their hands if they have socks or a belt on. Nearly everyone raises his or her hand. Then I ask them to lower their hands if they were not consciously aware of, or feeling, their socks or belt prior to me asking them to survey their bodies for the answer. Most of the people lower their hands at that point, because within moments of putting on socks, underwear, shirts, pants, belts, and the like, their brains recognized those sensory experiences as benign and quickly ignored the inputs. That process involves a phenomenon called *descending inhibition*, which is the release of inhibitory neurotransmitters onto the neurons in the brainstem that are receiving the input. (The peripheral nerves are not altered through this process, but the brain chooses to interpret the signals one way or another based upon an overall assessment of the circumstances. To this end, they say that paper cuts hurt eight times more when they occur at work versus when home relaxing.)

As the theory goes, if the brain has an expectation that an input is going to be benign, then the experience usually is less painful or even completely devoid of pain. Conversely, an expectation of pain leads to a reduction in the threshold for what can actually cause you to perceive an input as painful. So, how can the brain be programmed to have an expectation of pain that is abnormal (in either direction)? One way is for prior minor injuries to distort the proper interpretation of much more severe injuries. (The TED Talk by Lorimer Moseley of the University of South Australia is absolutely excellent on this topic, and it provides a very entertaining explanation of how the brain's expectations can cause completely erroneous [and even life-threatening] misperceptions of inputs.)

Another way to create the framework for inappropriate responses to inputs comes through chronic and/or severe activation of the immune system. In fact, this is how scientists often generate models of pain in animals. The animal models of migraine that Michael Oshinsky and Paul Durham created, which were presented in the discussion of headache, work in this way.

The way I describe this in presentations goes something like this:

Every cubic millimeter of your body has nerve endings that are constantly relaying information regarding the state of affairs in that little region up to the brainstem. The average timescale for these signals being sent is milliseconds, which means there are literally millions of bits of information streaming into the brain every second. The brain is organized to take in these bits of electrochemical data and to extract some meaning from them. At the highest level, the derived meaning could be "I have to go to the bathroom" or "The muscles in my legs are burning from this run," or "Darn, I can feel this cold is moving into my chest."

It turns out that a large portion of this autonomic data flooding the brainstem has to do with the immune system and energy production in the body (macrophages and mitochondria). Now, despite the fact that the immune system is always dealing with some level of viral and/or bacterial infection, the flow of information into the brainstem is typically muted by descending inhibition, and thus we don't consciously perceive those issues even though the immune system is working away in partnership with the nervous system to ensure we fight the small skirmish and recover. Mitochondrial function is not significantly disturbed, and all is well. In a sense, the brain runs a program that biases perception so the inputs it is receiving are deemed to be benign at the subconscious level (i.e., the biological equivalent of "dealing with this signal is below your pay grade").

Every once in a while, however, the autonomic nervous system sends signals that are strong enough to break through that descending inhibition muffler, and the signal is interpreted to be worthy of perception. The converse is also true, and occasionally the descending inhibition muffler weakens, and the signals that wouldn't otherwise have made it through to the world of perceptions show up. Anyone who has overindulged in alcohol has likely experienced this phenomenon the next morning when all forms of prior injuries mysteriously reappear because alcohol has the ability to degrade the natural pain filters that prevent you from experiencing the ongoing aches and pains from prior injuries or wear and tear.

Back to the example of the peripheral signals becoming strong enough to overcome normal descending inhibition. When this happens because of an immune problem (i.e., inflammation) the brain shifts into a different mode, which I refer to as a "sickness program." Interestingly, this program is designed to get you to change your behavior (e.g., to lie down, sleep, not eat, stay away from other people, and remain inactive). Now, it would be so much easier if the program simply gave you a voicemail that said these things, but it has no means for doing that. Plus, this is the same system that has to do the same thing for your dog or cat, so even texting won't work.

What it does, instead, is to make you tired, makes you a little dizzy and/or gives you a headache, lowers your mood, makes you nauseated, makes everything ache, and alters your metabolism and circadian rhythms so you can sleep for ten hours through the middle of the day. But here's the rub. If you think about it, these are the same symptoms that people with chronic fatigue, fibromyalgia, IBS, depression, migraine, and several other chronic conditions complain about, only they complain about them for years on end because they don't subside. Is it any wonder that they show up together at much higher than chance frequency and are very difficult to treat? The difference is, in the case of the flu, most people get over the symptoms, but it is very interesting that extended COVID-19 illness has been associated with a long-term condition, referred to as Long COVID, in which the symptoms mirror these chronic symptoms.

So, how does this persistent state in which the sickness program doesn't switch off come to be? The answer is a two-step process. The first step is a "real" inflammatory insult, and the second is a central change in the processing of inbound autonomic and sensory signaling. With respect to the first step, remember that physical, mental, and emotional threats can trigger inflammation. The insult(s) has to be prolonged and/or severe, and typically repeated. There are those who suggest that this first step of the process actually requires two insults that come in two different ways (i.e., a physical challenge followed by an emotional challenge). When the inflammation persists, it keeps the brain in the sick program for long enough that the descending inhibition and other mechanisms for properly categorizing inbound nerve impulses become dysfunctional. This becomes a vicious cycle as signals that are normally benign become triggers for further inflammatory responses peripherally and centrally. In a sense, you become sensitized to all inputs, at least of a certain type (e.g., severe or prolonged gastrointestinal inflammation leads to gastroparesis or IBS). This sensitization of the central nervous system, or central sensitization, is a form of maladaptive pain (and all autonomic signaling) processing.[164]

Clifford Woolf explains that pain, in a neuroimmunologic sense, can be broken down into *reactive* (to cause reflexive avoidance of threats like heat, sharpness, and pressure to minimize injury), *adaptive* (the lingering soreness of a bruise or burn, associated with the intermediate inflammatory response, that serves to limit use of the tissue during the repair period), and *maladaptive* (pain that is abnormal and serves no readily identifiable protective purpose) categories.[165] Reactive pain acts through pathways that pass through the spinal cord, limiting the need for higher processing. Adaptive pain activates areas (both sensory and emotional) in the central nervous system. The evolutionary purpose of this hypersensitivity pain is to promote healing and ensure that the individual does not aggravate the damage done by continued activity.

Maladaptive pain is further subdivided into two types: pain that arises from damage to the nervous system (e.g., neuropathic pain) and pain that comes as a result of improper functioning of the nervous system (dysfunctional pain). Central sensitization is dysfunctional and is often a consequence of inflammation that then becomes maladaptive as a result of the same neuro-immune responses described in chapter 2, like the degradation of descending inhibition, the release of factors like calcitonin gene-related peptide (CGRP). Thus, peripheral inflammation starts out as simple pain, but prolonged activation of these circuits creates an expectation of pain, and like a bike passing through the woods over and over again, single tracks become well-worn paths. Prolonged excitatory inputs from noxious signals create sensitized central circuits that remain chronically excited (i.e., in a pain state). Chronic pain leads from and to chronic inflammation, both resulting in a sensitization process within the CNS.

USE OF VNS IN MULTISYMPTOMATIC PATIENTS

As luck would have it, I was introduced to a group of clinical pharmacists in the UK who had access to hundreds of thousands of active patient files in electronic databases they could analyze. I explained to them what I needed, which was a set of patients who were severe headache sufferers and who were using a lot of healthcare resources. After a few weeks they showed me their preliminary findings. They had identified fifty patients with severe headache problems, and they had laid out all the healthcare-related expenses of these patients in a spreadsheet with their entire diagnostic, medical, and pharmaceutical prescription histories. It was actually far more information than I had expected to see about the patients, but I was immediately struck by something fascinating. The medical trajectories of these patients looked identical. They all had headaches, to be sure, but they also had multiple other conditions, starting with depression and/or anxiety, but also including sleep problems, allergies or asthma, GI problems, and many had widespread pain conditions ranging from endometriosis to fibromyalgia. Frankly, what I was seeing were the worst-case scenarios of what Pesa and Lage had written about more than a decade earlier, because the data now included far more than just mental health issues.

The interesting thing for me, of course, was that all of these conditions were ones for which VNS was being studied as a possible treatment. So, I had an idea. I asked the clinical pharmacist team to go out and not just focus on headache patients, but rather to provide me with a spreadsheet of ALL the diagnostic histories on ALL the patients in the various practices they had searched. They warned me that the spreadsheet would be massive, and they were right. The very first spreadsheet they sent me had over 150,000 lines of data. It crashed my computer about every fifteen minutes.

Sixteen hours later, however, I had uncovered something that was really remarkable. I had sorted all the patients into whether they had ever had any diagnoses for any of the conditions I had seen and read about, and therefore thought VNS might help treat. There were six condition "buckets": headache, depression or anxiety, gastric motility problems, sleep conditions, asthma or allergies (or chronic sinusitis), and widespread pain. Forty percent of the population in this group of thousands of patients had never been diagnosed with any of these conditions, and they seldom (if ever) went to their primary doctor, took medication, had trips to the hospital, or saw a specialist. Another 30 percent had been diagnosed with only one of the six conditions, and their costs (medication use, doctor's office visits, and trips to the hospital) were about the average. It was the next 30 percent, who had multiple diagnoses for these conditions, where things got interesting, and expensive. Incredibly, among a group of about 12 to 15 percent of the population who were simultaneously diagnosed with four, five, or even six of these conditions, the costs were off the charts.

Now, for those of you who are yawning about what I'm sharing, let me explain the punchline here. Let's say that the prevalence of each of these conditions is 10 percent, which is to say that one out of ten people has each of the medical problems I isolated (it's actually about 12 percent for migraine, but fibromyalgia is much lower at around 3 percent, GI problems is around

10 percent, and anxiety is even a bit higher than migraine, but 10 percent each is a good estimate to demonstrate my point). If one out of ten has migraine, and one out of ten has GI problems, then if these two problems aren't related, then the number of people who have both should be only 1 percent. Having three conditions should be a one in a thousand phenomenon. The data I was looking at showed that one in eight people had four or more conditions simultaneously. Something had to explain this outrageously higher level of comorbidity than statistics could account for.

Given that all of these conditions were ones that VNS treatments had either been approved to treat or there was clinical evidence supporting that it was likely to help, I set up a very simple study with the practices from whom we had gotten the original data. The goal was to see if VNS might work to help with all the symptoms the patients were experiencing simultaneously. To be accurate, the doctors didn't really even want to see these patients anymore, because they were in their offices all the time seeking care that never seemed to help. So, we compromised and said we'd invite the patients in to see the pharmacist to review their medications.

The doctors and the pharmacists told us that mass mailers would bring in about one or maybe two of these patients out of one hundred. Boy, were they wrong! Twenty percent of the people we wrote to showed up with the letter in their hands, asking how we knew that they experienced all of the symptoms we had listed. In most cases, the patients' records didn't even reflect all the symptoms, but the patients would typically explain that they had never gotten a diagnosis for some of the symptoms because they didn't want to have to take any more medications. They were just living with those symptoms untreated. When our pharmacists explained to the patients our thesis, that all of their symptoms might be related, and that there might be one underlying way to treat it, well, we had grown men tear up. Many responded with some form of, "I knew it, but nobody will listen." It was actually quite sad and frustrating to hear.

Intriguingly, many would continue, telling our pharmacists that their array of problems all stemmed from some single event in their lives (an illness, trauma, stressful life event, surgery, or emotional loss) and that in the aftermath of the event, they, "had not been the same since." It was easy to see how these people had lived through events that resembled what researchers were doing to animals in models of migraine and other conditions! Life was doing to these people what the researchers had figured out was the way to centrally sensitize animals.

We offered them our nVNS device to try and asked them to complete a simple five-question questionnaire every month that measured the basics of their quality of life. Literally 96 percent of the patients took us up on the offer. I'll tell you how they did in a minute, but first ...

While this study was taking off, I was introduced to another group in the UK, this time it was one that was actually part of the National Health System (the NHS), which is part of the government. This group keeps a searchable database that holds the medical records of over 6 million people, called the CPRD database. When I shared with the founder of the CPRD head, John Parkinson, what we were seeing, he was so taken that he had his team conduct the equivalent of about $300,000 worth of database analytics to confirm what our team of clinical pharmacists had found. When they produced the same results with their data, John Parkinson was blown away.

Meanwhile, during the three weeks per month that I was back here in the US, I was introduced to Dr. Timothy Smith, a neurologist who was running research for Mercy Health Systems. (Mercy Health Systems is the second-largest integrated health system in the country.) Being a headache neurologist by specialty, he did a quick review among the Mercy Health patients (across a group of 2 million patients) to find out how many who had migraine also had these other problems. What he found startled him tremendously: the most expensive subgroup of patients they had in their system was this group of multisymptomatic migraine patients. A group of 86,000 of them were costing $2 billion dollars per year. Worse yet, the costs for these patients were rising and because none of the conditions seemed to end (either in death or a cure), the lifetime costs of these patients exceeded any other group, including those with heart failure and cancer!

In the wake of these revelations, I decided to enlist the help of a data analytics firm called GNS Healthcare from Cambridge, Massachusetts. At the time, they had purchased access to a 100-million-patient database of private insurance healthcare costs across the US spanning a six-year period. I asked them to test the two theories:

1. Comorbidity across these six conditions were way outside the bounds of what might be randomly expected; and

2. The average costs of multisymptomatic patients are astronomically more expensive than average costs for everyone else. They had been proven in the UK as well

as in Mercy Health Systems, but the third time would be the charm. As expected, the results they came up with confirmed the findings.

The last bit of analytics we did was with one of the leading neurologists in the country, Dr. Richard Lipton, who is triple board certified and holds simultaneous positions in neurology, psychiatry, and epidemiology. Dr. Lipton had been a clinical study participant in the headache work that had been conducted to gain FDA clearance for the nVNS we had developed, and was, therefore, keenly interested in what I was looking into. When I shared with him the findings we had made from the original UK study, he realized that there was enough data in the spreadsheets to do what he referred to as a latent causation analysis, which is basically a mathematical test to determine if one of the conditions was driving all the other problems. The alternative, as Sherlock Holmes would have said, was that if there was no symptomatic condition driving the others, then the only alternative would be that an asymptomatic problem that was going undetected (or unappreciated) was underlying all the comorbidity. Of course, as you may have intuitively predicted, the latter is exactly what the analysis showed. Still, it left a big unanswered question, which was: What was the underlying problem that was this latent cause?

The question of what latent causes might be was one that Richard Lipton, himself, had been struggling with for more than a decade with respect to a narrower set of symptoms that arise out of migraine. In fairness, being interested in headache, he had focused a lot of his attention on the different features of migraine. I, on the other hand, was far more interested in the vagus nerve and the autonomic nervous system as a whole.

And so, I predicted that the problem was an autonomic nervous system imbalance that was leaving patients in a chronic sympathetically active state. As the reader has come to understand, sympathetic overdrive activates inflammation, making any attempt to treat a specific symptom challenging, and limits any benefits of medications that only mask them. That is, if the body is in a sympathetic state, getting better is like trying to climb a sheer rock face with no ropes or pitons. If the rest, digest, and restore mode can be induced, then the two most powerful forces in health (the nervous and immune systems) are working for you, and getting better will be a downhill slide.

Sure enough, when Richard Lipton asked his statisticians to analyze the data we had provided using this hypothesis, the patient data split right down the middle. Those with the autonomic nervous system dysfunctions had the symptoms, and those that didn't were largely free from the symptoms. As this answer was being revealed, a new question appeared: Can we reverse the central sensitization, or at least treat it, by modulating the autonomic nervous system? Now, the animal studies that Michael Oshinky and Paul Durham conducted had already provided us with hints, as had the clinical studies that we had conducted in headache and the work by others in depression, but doing a study across many seemingly different symptoms was not something researchers typically do.

The answer to that question returns us to the study of nVNS in the multisymptomatic patients in the UK. Not all of the patients adhered with treatment with the device we provided. In fact, we lost about a third of them the first month, but, in fairness, they hadn't gone to the visit expecting to enroll in a study. Many of the ones who did stick with it, however, started reporting back absolutely remarkable benefits across every aspect of their symptoms. The most consistent comments were around improved sleep, less pain (especially headaches), less anxiety, better mood, and better breathing. Some patients reported other benefits as well, including weight loss and better cognitive function. Most importantly, the improvement in the quality of life scores kept rising over the course of three months, and then maintained this high level for more than a year. The amount of improvement was about the same amount of improvement that people report with a total knee replacement (one of the most successful procedures in medicine), except the benefits weren't limited to mobility—they spanned the entire questionnaire.

CHAPTER 7

. . . .

EPIGENETICS, IMMUNE FUNCTION, AND THE VAGUS NERVE

Let's imagine that you have just been hired to run purchasing for the wildly popular 3-Michelin-star restaurant Chez Shells. The uber-famous head chef, Jacques St. Coquilles, has secretly written out, in code, his highly sought-after recipes for every mouthwatering dish on the menu. Your job is to buy the ingredients he will need to cook for all the customers who flock to his award-winning dining experience. As excited as you are to have landed this cushy job with amazing gustatory benefits, you quickly realize that the chef hasn't given you nearly enough information for you to do your job. Although he gave you the secret code to unlock what the ingredients are and how much of each ingredient goes into any given entrée, you have no idea how often patrons order each item. Should you buy more oxtail or duck? You also haven't a clue how long the John Dory on the list will last in the refrigeration locker, nor the Kobe beef flown in from Tokyo weekly. Finally, you don't know how demands change during the week, such as how many people are going to be dining on a Tuesday versus a Saturday.

Now imagine you are a nerve cell, sitting in the dorsal raphe nucleus (the major serotonin source in the brainstem) of Abigail, a thirty-five-year-old mother of twin nine-year-old boys, working in the back office of the Tampa Bay Rays. The team has just clinched a spot in tonight's wild card game, and Abby is waiting to see if she is going to be able to score an extra ticket from her boss, so she can take her twins to the game (leaving her husband home with the dog to watch the first game of the playoffs on television). You, the nerve cell inside Abigail's brainstem, are getting lots of signals from the other nerves around you that there could be a huge demand for serotonin coming up in the hours to come. To meet that demand, you are going to have to produce a lot of the protein (enzyme) tryptophan hydroxylase, or TPH. The good news is that you (along with every cell in the body you inhabit) have the coded instructions for how to make TPH. Of course, it is written in a gene somewhere among the three billion base pairs cut up into twenty-three pairs of chromosomes. The bad news is that the code is deeply buried inside a seemingly endless string of DNA that is balled up very tightly, bundled with literally millions of proteins. This means you are going to have to remember where that gene sits, and then find a way to unwind the code to get to the instructions for making TPH. Worse yet, whole sections of the code have been doused in glue, making it virtually impossible to unwind. If that weren't enough, there is a possibility that some other sections of the code, which look similar to key parts of the TPH gene, will oppose the production of the enzyme. Those may be produced at the same time you copy the gene you are looking for, and some of them are already floating around inside you, looking to prevent that TPH from being made ... that is, if you ever figure out how to copy the code.

If the two mental exercises above weren't dead giveaways, this chapter covers how cells know what genes to transcribe (and which ones to ignore), what proteins to manufacture, and how to ensure the right amount of each protein is made. After all, a nerve cell in the dorsal raphe nucleus has the same DNA with the same complement of genes that are in a hepatocyte in the liver, or a chondrocyte in the knee, or a cardiomyocyte in the heart. If every cell produced the protein from every gene, and the production of these proteins was constant across all cells in the body, there would be no such thing as differentiation of cells (in fact, it is highly unlikely that such a cell could even survive). There would also be a vastly more limited ability for the organism to alter its function in response to the environment around it.

What we are talking about is epigenetics, and more specifically, the epigenetic mechanisms of DNA methylation, histone modification, and non-coding RNAs that control whether genes in the DNA are transcribed into messenger RNA, transferred out of the nucleus to the ribosomes, and translated into proteins. Later in this chapter, we will also cover the topic of what is now termed *inflammaging*, the role of inflammation in affecting the pace at which our bodies age relative to the actual flow of time. I think it is fair to say that most people would be pleased to find a way to have their bodies age only one month for every year they are actually alive. While that is a very ambitious goal, and probably not a sustainable one over decades, by the end of this chapter, we'll discuss several key techniques to slow down the pace of aging so we and our descendants can live longer and healthier.

CONTROLLING DNA AND GENE EXPRESSION

Now, getting down to it, our story begins with one of those characters in the history of science whose theories were believed by many for decades, and then, in what seemed like a flash, abandoned and ridiculed, only to have his scientific legacy undergo a remarkable comeback centuries later. In this case, the man is Jean-Baptiste Lamarck (actually Jean-Baptiste Pierre Antoine de Monet, chevalier de Lamarck), and the resurgence of Lamarckian inheritance, at least certain aspects of it, has transpired within the past couple of decades.

More specifically, Lamarck was an 18th-century zoologist who proposed a theory of inheritance teaching that creatures are shaped by the demands of their environment. This is relatively uncontroversial when speaking of an individual animal, but Lamarck took the further step of hypothesizing that the changes induced by these environmental pressures were then passed on through inheritance to the creature's offspring. The classic example used by Lamarck was that of the giraffe's neck, which he claimed grew longer as each successive generation stretched to reach higher and higher leaves.

Students of Darwinian evolution may be cringing, and rightfully so; however, many are forgetting that Charles Darwin thought very highly of Lamarck's ideas. As a result of Darwin and Gregor Mendel (the German monk who was the father of genetic inheritance) and all the discoveries surrounding DNA that we are taught in high school, however, most people have come to the conclusion that physical attributes, like the neck length of giraffes, are determined solely by genes. But what do we mean by this? Are the genes that determine the makeup of neck bones in giraffes different from the neck bone genes of, say, the okapi (the only other member of the mammalian family *Giraffidae*), which do not have such profoundly long necks? The short answer (no pun intended) is no. It is not a stretch (sorry!) to say, however, that the determining factor for neck length is not (solely) in the genes themselves, but in how they are expressed, which, at an important level means the amounts of proteins that are made from various genes.

Evolution, which displaced Lamarck's theory, works like this: In an environment where food grows on high branches, animals who are lucky enough *to have* longer necks have a survival advantage, so they eat a lot and have babies. Short-necked giraffes have a disadvantage getting food and don't procreate as successfully, or they simply die off. So, long-necked giraffes survive, many reproduce with other long-necked giraffes, and violá, their children inherit genes for long necks. In a sense, evolution is a genetic arms race (or, in this case, a neck race). Longer necks keep reproducing until their necks are so long that a survival disadvantages start to kick in (like maintaining the pressure to get blood up a long neck to the brain). Frankly, that would have left giraffe necks a lot shorter if evolution had not solved that problem too (giraffes have special valves in their carotid arteries to help boost the pressure so blood can reach the brain).

But what about the okapi? They survived in the same environments in which giraffes evolved.

This is where you need to recall the explanation of genetics that I provided in chapter 1. As promised, I will provide a quick refresher here, but if you can't follow, please just jump back to chapter 1 for a page or two to refresh your recollection.

DNA is two strands of nucleic acids linked together vertically by a backbone of ribose (a sugar) and laterally, like rungs of a twisted ladder, through the pairings of matching nucleotide bases (adenine pairs with guanine, and cytosine pairs with thymine). In humans (and all eukaryotic life), DNA is contained in the nucleus of the cell where it is coiled around proteins called histones, and this coiled structure is then supercoiled further into tight packages called chromatin (yes, that's from the word chromosome) so that billions of base pairs can fit inside the tiny nucleus. Genes are stretches of DNA, sometimes broken up into distinct segments within the DNA, that are copied (transcribed) into messenger RNA (mRNA), which carry the message of how a specific protein is to be constructed. mRNA leaves the nucleus and travels to a protein manufacturing machine called a ribosome. The mRNA strand is then written (translated) into a protein.

Stretches of DNA slightly upstream from the genes (or gene parts) themselves are referred to as promoter sequences. These sequences promote the binding of other proteins to the DNA to initiate the unwinding and copying processes. More specifically, the highly coiled, super-tightly wound DNA must be unpacked, or unwound, from the histones so it can be "unzipped" and copied into RNA, after which it can be re-zipped and repacked. Deciphering the elaborate steps necessary to coordinate this transcription process over the past eighty years has revealed miraculous ways in which protein expression is regulated. What makes these control mechanisms so remarkable is that they can be modulated by the environment and the life experiences of the individual animal, and as we will see later, they may be *inherited* by the next generation, just as Lamarck suggested could happen!

EPIGENETICS

So, let's dive into epigenetics, which Google (as of this writing) defines as:

> The study of how your behaviors and environment can cause changes that affect the way your genes work. Unlike genetic changes, epigenetic changes are reversible and do not change your DNA sequence, but they can change how your body reads a DNA sequence.

To be honest, some epigenetic changes may not be reversible, at least not in your lifetime, and some can actually lead to mutations in your DNA. As for the part about changing "how your body reads a DNA sequence," a better way to say it might be changing "when and how a DNA sequence can be accessed." More specifically, certain genes are only necessary during growth in utero, or only up through puberty, or just during or in the period after pregnancy, and still others are critical for viability at any age. Turning genes on or off, temporarily or permanently, is a very important function of epigenetics.[166] Epigenetic modification of protein expression makes all of life far more flexible, robust, and capable of surviving challenges.

As suggested by the example of the neuron in the dorsal raphe nucleus of the mother of twin Tampa Bay Rays fans, there are two primary ways to epigenetically control protein expression. The first is to prevent the gene from being copied into mRNA. The second is to prevent the copied mRNA from being used as the template for making protein.[167] All three of the mechanisms described below have the ability to do the first. Non-coding RNA, which is the third of these to be described, is the one primarily responsible for the latter.

DNA METHYLATION

The first mechanism of epigenetic control over gene transcription is DNA methylation, which has roots that pre-date the discovery of DNA.[168] In 1925, Johnson and Coghill discovered a chemically altered form of the nucleotide base, cytosine, that had the ability to keep DNA in its coiled structure and to resist unwinding for transcription. Recall that copying of a gene into RNA requires that transcription factors have access to the DNA sequence. Changing the tightness of the coiling can bury what was an exposed promoter sequence or the gene itself deep inside the wound structure.

To understand how DNA methylation works, recall how DNA is stored. Proteins called histones serve as spools around which the DNA is wrapped, and these histones associate to form a unit called a nucleosome. A single unit normally associates with a sequence of approximately 147 base pairs of DNA. Series of these units are linked together by a different type of histone.[169] This organization offers protection of the DNA against damage and serves as the substrate for multiple mechanisms that regulate access to the genes. Methylation of DNA alters the fundamental structure of the nucleosome, shifting the number of base pairs wrapped around a unit, which shifts the location of promoter-binding regions, so they are no longer accessible. Chemical modification of the DNA also changes its electrical charge in a way that changes how easily the histone releases it for transcription.

DNA methylation is facilitated by a naturally occurring class of enzymes called DNA methyltransferases, or DNMTs. These proteins are often referred to as "writers" leaving "marks" on the DNA. Similarly, other proteins "read" the marks and become attached to the site, therein amplifying the effects, including blocking access to the DNA wrapped around histones.[170] (Recall the reference to the glue being poured over the bundled DNA in the story of the neuron at the beginning of the chapter.) DNMT writers typically methylate cytosines that are adjacent to guanine along the same side of the DNA sequence, in what is generally referred to as a CpG dinucleotide (CpG stands for cytosine-phosphate-guanine).

In addition to tighter wrapping of DNA around histones, methylated CpGs serves as a site where special proteins associate with the DNA to physically shield it from other proteins programmed to copy the gene.

Thinking statistically, in a genome of 3 billion base pairs, random chance would dictate that one in four bases is a cytosine (and it is actually 24 percent in humans). Similarly, one in four of those cytosines would be followed by a guanine (with a phosphate between), meaning that CpGs (again, this is not across the ladder as a single rung but along one side of the ladder) should randomly occur at approximately one out of sixteen dinucleotides. In DNA that contains 3 billion base pairs, that means there have to be at least 360 million CpGs. How does the cell know which cytosines to methylate?

First, it turns out that CpGs are relatively rare in the eukaryotic genome, especially among higher animals. Humans, for example, have only about 28 million CpGs, meaning CpGs appear less than 10 percent of the time that would otherwise be expected. (Curiously, in bacteria, the frequency of CpG is closer to the level expected through random occurrence.) The fact is that cytosines are relatively easy to methylate and are readily deaminated into thymine under physiological conditions. This can result in a point mutation in the DNA that permanently alter the genetic sequence, which would be a major issue for genetic integrity. Thus, natural selection has seen to it that CpGs have been systematically removed from the genome to minimize this risk. This phenomenon is referred to as *CpG Suppression*, but it is not a suppression in any active sense that the DNA has been purposefully cleansed of CpGs. It is just the result of millions of generations of creatures surviving better with less mutation risk.[171]

In fact, the percentage of CpG dinucleotides in the gene-containing portions of eukaryotic DNA is even lower than the approximately 10 percent cited above. This is because the one exception to this rule of reduced CpG frequency exists in areas called *CpG islands*. CpG islands are defined as stretches of at least 200 base pairs, in which at least 50 percent of the dinucleotides are CpG, which is fifty times the average frequency in the genome. These islands occur in close proximity to promoter sequences, and, in fact, about 60 percent of promoters have CpG islands associated with them. Methylation of many of the cytosines in CpG islands leads to a change in the helical tilt of the DNA, a significant tightening of the winding of the DNA around histones. The practical upshot is that methylated genes are typically being shielded from being accessed.[172]

That rule is not absolute, because about 5 percent of the CpG islands are associated with enhancer sequences, which are used to keep DNA unwound and exposed for easy transcription. In this situation, DNA methylation is like the deadbolt that can be extended when the door is open, to keep it from closing. That's what happens when CpG islands in the vicinity of enhancer sequences are methylated. These islands are typically shorter (e.g., 50 to 150 base pairs in length, compared with the promoter sequence islands, and are referred to as *orphan CpG islands*.)[173] This is a break from the general rule, but certainly an important exception.

For a long time, methylation was considered to be irreversible, but it is now known that, in addition to writers and readers, there are also "erasers" (a group of several versions are collectively called ten-eleven translocators, or TETs) that can remove the methylation mark. Interestingly, the activity of erasers is tightly regulated and is seen during developmental stages when cells that were previously fully differentiated need to undergo new changes. Examples of this occur during puberty, during pregnancy (e.g., the creation of lactating tissue in breasts), and in aging. Pathological conditions in which demethylation occurs include migraine, pain chronification,* and cancer.[174]

The existence of writers, like DNMTs, and erasers, like TETs, is evidence that DNA methylation is a dynamic process happening to DNA, which had previously been considered relatively

---

* Pain chronification is the neurological shift from experiencing pain as an acute response to injury, or even a lingering sensation coupled with the healing process, to a permanent state of pain associated with a change in the interpretation of nerve impulses from an affected region of the body.

static. While genes may be fixed, epigenetic mechanisms, like DNA methylation, serve as a means for the environment and the actual experiences and activities of an organism to affect their genes, or at least the expression levels of those genes. Lamarck meets Darwin!

Some of the life events and circumstances that have been studied relative to DNA methylation are food scarcity (starvation), mental and physical abuse, war, and overnutrition (obesity). Each of these situations is associated with stress, the production of reactive oxygen species, and inflammation, which collectively have been blamed for the process of aging. DNA methylation has, thus, also been extensively studied in aging, to the point that changes in methylation states across hundreds of thousands of sites within the human genome can now be used to predict physiologic age and even the rate of aging. As will be seen later in this chapter, DNA methylation and other epigenetic factors explain some of the features of the Mitochondrial Theory of Aging,[175] which holds that progressive damage to mitochondria, and increased leakage of ROS, breaks down organs and leads to an increase in inflammation that degrades our bodies until we become less resilient and unable to recover, and ultimately, die.

More specifically, aging and damage to the methylome (the term used to describe the entirety of the DNA methylation state) are associated with a combination of methylation, demethylation, and collective damage from ROS. For example, demethylation has been observed in pathways that perceive stress and/or pain, as pain sensing and processing neurons function differently in the aftermath of severe or chronic pain, leading to the development of neuropathic pain. This means that blocking of demethylation and/or the enhancement of methylation activity, depending on the gene affected, can actually reduce chronified pain.[176]

Eukaryotic cells can be categorized by the level to which they are differentiated. For example, adipose cells and hepatocytes are fully differentiated, while progenitor cells are the stem cells that produce new, more differentiated cells, as needed. Climbing back up to the top of the food chain of cells leads to germline cells (i.e., sperm and eggs). Somatic cells are the differentiated cells, and the purpose of DNA methylation within these cells is relatively obvious. Protein expression in such cells is limited to specific purposes, but because the demands of the environment can fluctuate, the varying levels of this limited number of proteins depend on circumstances.

In germ-line cells, DNA has to start out with very few methylation marks, but must slowly rebuild the marks that are required as development progresses. It turns out that sperm tend to have their methylation marks stripped more effectively than eggs, meaning that the father's genetic contribution is more available, but the other mother's serves as a template for replacing the DNA methylation marks as the individual develops. This turns out to be very important, also, for the passage of epigenetic marks that are the result of environmental pressures. It has been hypothesized, and strong animal data support the conclusion, that life experiences of parents, grandparents, and even great-grandparents (at least those experiences that occurred prior to bearing children) can be imprinted through epigenetics. To date, however, the evidence for epigenetic inheritance through DNA methylation remains controversial.

In a first case, Heijmans and colleagues studied the genomes of individuals and their offspring who had survived the Dutch Hunger Winter of 1944 to 1945. In their paper, published in *Nature Communications*, titled "DNA methylation signatures link prenatal famine exposure to growth and metabolism," the authors reported that the offspring who had been exposed to maternal starvation-level diets in early gestation had statistically significant alterations in their DNA methylation of multiple genes associated with development and metabolism. These offspring experienced (paradoxically) higher birth weights than babies born either before that period or after, at the same hospitals. In addition, they evidenced a higher predisposition to several aspects of metabolic syndrome, including higher BMI, lipid dysregulation, and altered glucose metabolism.[177]

Similarly, Yehuda and colleagues analyzed a small cohort of Holocaust survivors and their offspring, looking at methylation at a gene (FKBP5) associated with PTSD symptoms.[178] In their findings, the survivors showed a 10 percent higher rate of methylation of the gene, while their offspring had a nearly 8 percent reduction in its methylation, and were more prone to depression, anxiety, and PTSD symptoms than matched controls.

HISTONE MODIFICATION

As stated previously, multiple histones form the structural unit that DNA is wound around. In fact, there are eight histones, two each of histones H2A, H2B, H3, and H4, that form that unit. The hold that these proteins have on the DNA wrapped around them isn't overly strong, so the energy required to expose DNA is low.

Modification of even a single amino acid of a histone can alter its binding affinity for DNA, altering binding tightness and altering the topology and accessibility to promoter sequences.[179]

Histones can be modified by several chemical changes, including acetylation, methylation, deamination, phosphorylation, and ubiquitination, to its amino acids.[180] Generally, these involve an alteration of a side group of one or more peptides located at the end of the peptide sequence that has been wound up tightly into a ball, called the "tail." These alterations are referred to as post-translational modifications (or PTMs), and like DNA methylation, which is mediated by DNMTs, these reactions are catalyzed by histone-modifying enzymes. The full list of possible post-translational modifications of histones is beyond the scope of this book, but we will focus on two common examples, which are acetylation and methylation, and which are mediated by histone acetyltransferases (HATs) and histone methyltransferases (HMTs), respectively.

In the case of acetylation, an HAT typically attaches an acetyl group to a lysine (an amino acid with a charged polar sidechain). Nearly universally, the addition of the acetyl group reduces the electrostatic forces binding the DNA to the histone, and thus is associated with loosening the grip of the DNA on the histone, making unwinding easier for transcribing the gene. Histone deacetylase proteins reverse the process, often after transcription is complete and it is time to store the DNA away again. For obvious reasons, these are extremely important functions, and more than thirty separate HAT proteins have been identified. Dysregulation of histone acetylation has been associated with cancer and other serious medical conditions.[181]

Histone 3 has lysines located at the 4th, 9th, and 27th positions of its tail (abbreviated H3K4, H3K9, and H3K27, where K is the single letter code for lysine). These amino acids are consistently associated with upregulation and downregulation of gene expression. In contrast to acetylation, which typically promotes transcription, these same histone locations can be methylated. In fact, methylation can involve a single methyl group (monomethylated, or me1), two groups (dimethylated, or me2), or three (trimethylated, or me3).[182]

Another variable that affects protein expression is the location of the gene within the chromosomal structure. The location of genes relative to the center or ends of the chromosomal structure influences its expression. In fact, genes in these two locations are generally silent after development. This stable silencing is typically associated with histone deacetylation and trimethylation (i.e., H3K9me3). [183]

Let's dig into the various methylation sites and what effects they have. Starting with the simplest, H3K4 methylation is typically associated with actively transcribed genes.[184] (This promotion of transcription is enabled by a complex of proteins called COMPASS.[185]) The general rule of thumb developed by Sharifi-Zarchi and colleagues is:

> In each genomic region only one out of these three methylation marks {DNA methylation, H3K4me1, H3K4me3} is high. If it is the DNA methylation, the region is inactive. If it is H3K4me1, the region is an enhancer, and if it is H3K4me3, the region is a promoter.[186]

Next, H3K9 methylation has a more complicated activity, often dependent upon factors ranging from the mechanism and number of the methylation, to the level of reactive oxygen species (ROS). For example, H3K9me3 is associated with heterochromatin protein 1 (HP1) complexes that inhibit the unwinding of the DNA for transcription.[187]

Now, H3K27 is a bit more complicated. In general, H3K27me is typically associated with the slightly more flexible packing of DNA between the central and end portions of the chromosome. In this region of the chromatin, H3K27me3 associates with a group of proteins that work together as polycomb repressive complex (specifically PRC2). This association is dependent on a properly functioning DNA methylome. It also interacts with H3K9me3 to maintain HP1 engaged with the chromatin. Thus, H3K27me3 usually inhibits expression. As explained by Luciano Di Croce and colleagues in 2020, "PRC2 mediates gene repression through direct interaction with its target genes and deposition of the repressive H3K27me3 mark." If there are mutations in the histone gene, failure to properly methylate H3K27 can lead to a failure to repress genes, which can lead to childhood cancers as proteins that should no longer be expressed start to be.[188]

In contrast to trimethylation at this site, H3K27me1 (monomethylation) is associated with genes that will be expressed for some period of time, but then be turned off. H3K27me1 accumulates within transcribed genes, especially in stem cells that have yet to differentiate, promoting transcription. Once the cell terminally differentiates and requires gene repression, PCR2 then promotes further methylation.[189] H3K27me2 (dimethylation) can serve as an intermediate between H3K27me1 and H3K27me3, as a more flexible state of accessibility, but once the H3K27me3 is reached, the gene is typically shut off.

Histone modification affects diseases in extremely complicated ways; however, in a 2022 paper by Xiabin Chen and colleagues, the authors described the effects of histone methylation in the development and progression of atherosclerosis. According to their research:

> Methylation of H3K9 and H3K27 was decreased in atherosclerosis plaques in smooth muscle cells (SMCs), and H3K4 methylation showed a significant association with the severity of atherosclerosis. Besides, histone H3K27 trimethylation could be catalyzed by PRC2 with EZH2, which is deemed to increase macrophage inflammatory responses. A recent study showed that EZH2-deficient mice reduced the levels of H3K27me3 and decreased H3K27 methyltransferase activity and also showed a significant reduction of lesion size suggesting the improvement of atherosclerosis.[190]

These findings in atherosclerosis, which we know from chapter 3 is an inflammatory condition, are a natural segue to the effects that inflammation and oxidative stress have on histone modification. Recent evidence indicates that the presence of inflammation leads to histone acetylation and promotional methylation of histones (H3K27me1), enhancing gene expression and leading to perpetuation of inflammatory cytokine expression. This observation has been made especially with respect to microglia.[191]

This is similar to what was previously described as the effect of aging.[192] Unlocking the expression of genes that have been previously suppressed, for example because they are no longer needed (e.g., associated with gestational or early childhood development), can be quite disruptive to homeostasis later in life. An important example that may play a critical role in Alzheimer's disease is the dysregulation of "eat me" and "don't eat me" signaling that can occur among senescent microglia.

Looking at the relationship between oxidative stress and histone modification, the two appear to exert bidirectional control on one another.[193] The bidirectionality relates to both whether the effects are to increase or decrease protein expression, as well as whether the histone modification is caused by, or affects, the level of reactive oxygen species. In both cases, these bidirectional influences can be oppositional, perhaps driving a stable equilibrium. For example, increases in the expression of an important mitochondrial antioxidant called superoxide dismutase (or SOD) that reduces ROS can reduce H3K9me3. Similarly, H3K9me3 demethylation prevents the activation of ROS production triggered by matrix metalloproteinase-9 (MMP-9), which is known for having pro-ROS effects in mitochondria.[194]

While there is this bidirectional control of histone methylation with respect to ROS generation, there appears to be an inexorable increase in mitochondrial stress and inflammation with time. This slide toward oxidative stress and inflammatory damage is likely a key player in the initiation and development of a spectrum of long-term conditions that appear in aging.[195] There are, however, some tantalizing hints that epigenetic manipulation may have positive effects on longevity. Epigenetic modification may be a key answer to some of humanity's biggest health challenges, aging among them.

Before shifting gears to the third major mechanism of epigenetics, microRNA (and other small RNA so-called non-coding sequences), we return to the subject of intergenerational and transgenerational inheritance. Unlike DNA methylation, histone modification is an established mechanism for extra-genetic transmission of protein expression control across generations. In order for these modifications to be inherited, two mechanisms must be present.[196]

The first is a mechanism that ensures histones are reincorporated into the daughter DNA (the products of the replication) at or near their positions in the parent DNA. Digging into this we find that, after DNA replication, nucleosomes are generally divided equally between the two daughter chromosomes, and the location of histones relative to the specific sequences is quite stable over many cell divisions. There is a suggestion of the existence of histone chaperones that associate with the DNA replication protein complexes (DNA polymerases) to ensure these marks are reproduced.[197] Provided the histones have not been otherwise stripped of their prior modifications, half of the nucleosomes of each daughter chromosome will retain the modifications of the original complement of DNA because the same altered histones will slide back into place in the daughter DNA.

The second mechanism required to ensure the reintroduction of the histone modifications after DNA replication on the daughter DNA with new histones, is a "read-write" complex that reads histone modification placement on one and writes on the other. More specifically, this complex could either read the histone modifications on one daughter chromosome and write the modifications onto the other daughter, or it could read the modifications of the original (parent) nucleosome and recruit a writer to follow with the daughter that does not retain the original histones and modify the new nucleosomes. Although more complicated, the latter has been more readily identified. Read-write mechanisms of the sort just described have been identified for H3K9 and H3K27[198] methylation.

Unlike H3K9 and H3K27 methylation, reincorporation of H3K4 methylation isn't as faithfully reproduced because it is associated with regions of chromosomes where a lot of the variation in gene expression occurs during life. That doesn't mean there isn't a mechanism; it's just different, and it is based on whether the gene was being actively transcribed prior to the cell dividing. That is, if the gene was unwound for transcription, that section of DNA containing the gene is translated to a location near the periphery of the nucleus. From this location, the DNA interacts with a structure referred to as the *nuclear pore complex*. During replication, the parent and daughter DNA sections will still remain in close proximity to the nuclear pore complex, and that leads to H3K4me2 modification. This form of methylation leaves the gene in a partially repressed state that can be rapidly deployed. Some authors refer to this as a "poised" state (i.e., repressed but available at a moment's notice).[199] This permissive state caused by the physical proximity to the nuclear pore complex survives through several generations in single-celled animals. Evidence for similar inheritance in complex multicellular life has yet to emerge. Of course, if the gene is not in that location, it is trimethylated, making it more securely repressed.

NON-CODING RNAS

Unlike prokaryotes, which have a much denser organization of a much smaller set of genes (usually a loop of DNA containing a few hundred to a couple thousand genes), eukaryotic genes account for only 1 to 2 percent of nuclear DNA. (Makes you wonder why we even call it a genome if that is the case?) This, it turns out, is a big clue that there is more coded into DNA than just genes. Of course, there are RNA structures that do jobs, like transfer RNA (a.k.a. tRNAs), which transport amino acids to ribosomes and match codons to peptides. In the human genome, there are some 500 copies of DNA sequences that code for tRNAs,[200] but this is a tiny fraction of the remainder.

What purpose, therefore, does the rest of the DNA serve? It turns out that in higher species, like humans, much of our DNA is comprised of regulatory sequences that control gene expression. Included in this vast category are microRNAs (miRNA), short-interfering RNA (siRNA), and PIWI-interacting RNA (piRNA), all of which serve critical roles in epigenetic modification of mRNA expression. Collectively, these molecules are referred to as RNAi. Associated with these special RNA is a group of proteins called argonautes. Argonautes are actually divided into two general groups, the AGO proteins and the PIWI proteins. Each has the ability to bind with an RNA sequence to form a complex called the RNA-induced silencing complex (RISC) to silence protein expression at the ribosome.[201] PIWI proteins have additional functions that will be discussed later in the chapter.

Starting with miRNA, these sequences begin as segments of RNA as long as 70 to 100 nucleotides or more. They have two special properties. First, they are very similar to protein coding genes (in fact, they are often partially transposed fragments of the original gene). Second, their sequence is partially complementary, or self-binding.[202] A short example might be:

GTCGTAG<u>AGTGA</u>**GTC**TTAAGTAC**AGA**TCAATG**CTAAGT**CATTGA
ATG<u>GTACTTAA</u>**ACT**<u>TCACTC</u>GCTTGA

Note that the sequence can be doubled over on itself as shown below to demonstrate complementarity.

GTCGTAG<u>AGTGA</u>**GTC**<u>TAGTAC</u>**AGA**<u>TCAATG</u>**CTA**

<u>AGTTCG</u><u>CTCACT</u>**TCA**<u>ATCATG</u>**GTA**<u>AGTTAC</u>**TGA**

You can see that the straight underlined areas form pairs of nucleotides that complement one another, meaning that they could be stable in a double helix form, provided the dotted underlined portion turned like a hairpin acts like a hinge. Even though the two ends don't align with the other bolded areas, the overall compatibility of the straight underlined areas is enough to hold the double-stranded RNA stable.

This RNA sequence, called the primary transcript for obvious reasons, which is doubled over on itself, is then captured by a protein called DROSHA (or its analog PASHA[203]). DROSHA proteins clip off the (uncolored) overlapping ends that are meaningless and cut the ribose backbone of the RNA at the strained hairpin turn.

<u>GAGTGA</u>**GTC**<u>TAGTAC</u>**AGA**<u>TCAATG</u>**CTA**

<u>CTCACT</u>**TCA**<u>ATCATG</u>**GTA**<u>AGTTAC</u>**TGA**

Next, the pre-miRNA is transported out of the nucleus by Exportin-5. Once outside the nucleus, the pre-miRNA is again captured by a protein, this time called DICER,[204] which clips off the former hairpin turn section (yellow), leaving a pair of mostly complementary RNA segments that are between twenty-one and twenty-four nucleotides long.

GAGTGA**GTC**TAGTAC**AGA**TCAATG

CTCACT**TCA**ATCATG**GTA**AGTTAC

The final step in the process is when the argonaute protein, AGO, grabs the sequence, untwists the double helix structure, separates the two largely complementary strands, and discards one while holding on to the other. (The one it lets go is quickly degraded as most unchaperoned genetic material outside the nucleus is broken down.) The AGO and miRNA quickly associate with another set of proteins which collectively form the RNA-induced silencing complex, or RISC. The RISC complex is brought to the ribosomes, and when it finds a messenger RNA sequence that it is a partial match for, the microRNA binds to (and sometimes even cuts) the messenger RNA sequence, gumming up the protein synthesis process.[205]

Short, or small, interfering RNA (siRNA) are virtually identical in how they are processed and what they do. The only real difference is that they are slightly longer (twenty-four nucleotides).[206]

PIWI-interacting RNA, however, are quite different. The RNA of many piRNAs is sourced from long single-stranded RNA, transcribed from regions of the DNA that have previously been considered "junk." Clusters of hundreds of piRNA sequences have been found in the DNA, often near the centromere, in the heterochromatin. The strands of piRNA, after being trimmed (by the ZUC-processor complex) are typically twenty-four to thirty-three nucleotides in length. piRNA are functionally similar in some respects to miRNA and siRNA, but instead of associating with AGO proteins, the RNA in piRNA associate with PIWI proteins. Also, unlike miRNA and siRNA, both of which are dominant in all cell types, piRNA are primarily used in germline cells because they have an ability to protect germline cells from changes to the genome.[207] This domain of importance is related to piRNA's ability regulate both transcription and translation.

Let's break that last bit down, because it is extremely important. piRNA is an RNA-induced silencing complex (piRISC) that serves as both a ribosomal and/or nuclear regulatory element. So it modulates the expression of genes at multiple locations. First, as with miRNA and siRNA, piRNAs interact with messenger RNA sequences at ribosomes. Unlike miRNA and siRNA, however, piRNAs can also interact directly and target DNA in the nucleus, silencing transcription (through DNA methylation and histone modification). This means piRNAs exert both translational and transcriptional control over protein expression. More specifically with respect to this transcriptional control, in germline cells, piRNA have the ability to target sequences of DNA referred to as transposons, which can unleash havoc on germline DNA, typically eliminating the viability of offspring.[208]

To say that piRNA are important is putting it mildly. For a perspective, there are only a few thousand miRNAs and siRNAs that have been identified. Compared with a genome that contains an estimated 20 to 25,000 genes, we could consider them a bit of an afterthought (of course, that's not true functionally, but from a percentage of the genome perspective, you see my point). In contrast, more than 173 million possible piRNAs have been identified (their coding sequences in the DNA can even overlap one another).[209] This makes piRNA the biggest player in genetics, again, from a percentage of the overall DNA package standpoint. As a group, they have to be that massive if they are going to be capable of interacting with unpredictable sequences, such as erroneous repeats, which, as their names suggest, are sections of repeated DNA (typically short sections repeated many times). piRNA also interact and silence transposons, which are stretches of DNA with the ability to move (or "jump") to distal positions within the genome.

Collectively making up nearly half of the genome, the majority of repeated elements are classified as short and long interspersed elements, comprising approximately 20 percent and approximately 17 percent of the human genome, respectively. These mistakes are the second and third biggest chunks of the total DNA! Conditions ranging from Huntington's Chorea (a devastating neurological condition that arises from an expansion of short repeat elements) to strong predispositions to forms of cancer are associated with erroneous repeats.

Originally discovered by Barbara McClintock, for which she won the Nobel Prize, transposons are sections of DNA that have the ability to move from one location to another within the DNA. There are two mechanisms by which these sections move: 1. the direct movement of a sequence of nucleotides from one location to another (referred to as "cut and paste") and 2. the transcription of an RNA intermediate that leads to a reverse transcription back to DNA that is then inserted into a new location within the genome (referred to as "copy and paste"). Transposons likely exist in the genome as lingering remnants of past viral encounters with the genomes of our ancestors, and some theorize that they remain because they can enhance the ability of a species, as a whole, to create effective mutations when it confronts a serious challenge (that epigenetics can't address).[210] However, for an individual trying to reproduce, transposons typically block viability of offspring because they shift the location of a critical gene, or a part of a gene, or insert a big chunk of nonsense right in the middle of another gene. PIWI proteins and several effector proteins that interact with the piRNA complex, therefore, have the ability to activate histone modification proteins like histone methyltransferases specific for H3K9me3 which silence the transposon. piRNA prevent the chaos of jumping genes from ensuing.

NON-CODING RNA AND OXIDATIVE STRESS

With this understanding of ncRNA, we can switch to a discussion of inflammation and oxidative stress, and how they interact with the functioning of non-coding RNA. Previously, it was explained that ROS (reactive oxygen species) play an important role in cellular health, with their involvement as signaling molecules for mitochondrial communication within the cell being critical to the maintenance of homeostasis, but excessive ROS levels being damaging and toxic. miRNAs play an important role in regulating cellular ROS level, and dysregulation of their levels can lead to oxidative stress and development of many medical conditions.[211] This relationship is bidirectional inasmuch as increased inflammation and oxidative stress imposed on the cell by exogenous threats and proinflammatory signaling alter miRNA (and siRNA) expression.

More specifically, with respect to the role of miRNA influence over ROS-mediated oxidative stress and damage to tissue, in 2017, Jaideep Banerjee and colleagues provided an excellent overview of important examples of medical conditions affected by the relationship between miRNA and oxidative stress.[212] Their review of the literature highlighted:

- Atherosclerosis and vascular disease,
- Heart attack,
- Type 2 diabetes,
- Cancer,
- Chronic kidney disease (CKD),
- Fatty liver disease, and
- Aging.

Beginning with atherosclerosis, the authors of this editorial review, entitled *MicroRNA Regulation of Oxidative Stress*, describe the role of a specific miRNA-210 in the protection of endothelial cells against oxidative stress-induced apoptosis. Protection provided by enhanced miRNA-210 expression is through its inhibitory effect on damaging ROS levels. Recall that higher levels of ROS can lead to cell suicide through a mitochondrially mediated caspase-activating pathway, so reduced ROS is a cell survival pathway. miRNA-210 regulates the oxidative damage to endothelial cells in other vascular conditions, as well.

In a similar way, in type 2 diabetes, higher levels of miRNA-424 is associated with lower expression levels of inflammatory cytokines like Il-1 and IL-6. In stroke models, another miRNA, let7A, is associated with the maintenance of integrity of the blood-brain barrier (and the reduction in inflammatory response and cell death). In each of these conditions, these observations of miRNA expression changes can be associated with vagus nerve stimulation.

As mentioned above, the relationship is bidirectional, and oxidative stress can alter the expression of miRNA. This point was driven home by Andrii Domanskyi and colleagues in their 2019 paper:

> MicroRNA networks and oxidative stress are inextricably entwined in neurodegenerative processes. Oxidative stress affects expression levels of multiple microRNAs and, conversely, microRNAs regulate many genes involved in an oxidative stress response. Both oxidative stress and microRNA regulatory networks also influence other processes linked to neurodegeneration, such as mitochondrial dysfunction, deregulation of proteostasis, and increased neuroinflammation, which ultimately lead to neuronal death.[213]

As the authors describe, a series of insults, ranging from insulin signaling dysregulation to amyloid-β aggregates contribute to mitochondrial dysfunction and oxidative stress. Associated with these physiologic phenomena are changes in miRNA expression. Oxidative stress causes both up- and downregulation of different miRNAs and, conversely, many microRNAs can regulate oxidative stress response.

HOW VNS AFFECTS EPIGENETIC MECHANISMS

Between 2005 and 2010, multiple research teams published results showing an interaction between immune function and miRNA. miRNA can modulate the expression of receptors and cytokines involved in immune responses, and changes in miRNA expression are associated with cytokine-triggered and/or LPS-induced inflammation. Tili, Pedersen, and their respective colleagues published data in 2007 showing that miRNA, including miRNA-155 and miRNA-146a, are upregulated by inflammatory triggers and play a role in CNS inflammation. Thus, collectively, these reports suggest at least these two miRNAs form feedback control mechanisms to blunt the effects of the proinflammatory triggers.[214]

In 2009, with knowledge of the newly proposed mechanisms of the CAP, which utilizes VNS to induce acetylcholine release, which acts to reduce inflammation, a group in Israel hypothesized that miRNA might play a role in this phenomenon. In animal studies published in *Immunity*, by Soreq and colleagues, microRNA-132 was shown to be upregulated by vagus nerve stimulation, and that miRNA-132 repressed the expression of enzyme acetylcholine esterase, which rapidly breaks down acetylcholine.[215] (Acetylcholine esterase is induced by stress.) Thus, VNS mediates an increase in acetylcholine by inhibiting the production of the enzyme that breaks it down.

Subsequent studies in stroke models confirmed the role of miRNA-132 in reducing the inflammatory response to ischemia and limiting the lesion size. That is, miRNA-132 was protective against the neuron-damaging inflammatory response to hypoxic injury in the brain.[216] As was previously described in chapter 2, VNS has been shown to provide similar benefits in animal models of stroke, and nVNS is currently being studied in human trials in Europe.

In 2015, Jiang and colleagues reported on similar work conducted in China showing that the antioxidant and anti-apoptosis benefits of VNS in an ischemia and reperfusion model of stroke were mediated through the upregulation of miRNA-210.[217] In fact, in their model, blocking of the miRNA-210 substantially eliminated the benefits of VNS!

Another microRNA that has been associated with the cholinergic anti-inflammatory pathway is miRNA-124. Levels of miRNA-124 have been shown to be increased in LPS-induced inflammatory models coupled with an agonist of α7-nAChR. According to further work by Soreq, published with Nadorp in 2014, miRNA-124 affects two proteins in the VNS-activated CAP.[218] These are:

1. STAT3, the reduction of which affects an inhibition of IL-6, and

2. TNFα converting enzyme, which reduces the release of TNFα.

miRNA-124 is highly expressed in the mammalian brain, conferring stress resilience, and is downregulated in the hippocampus of stressed animals. Animal models of traumatic brain injury (TBI) have shown a curious transient rise in miRNA-124, followed by a decrease associated with an elevation in neurodegenerative risk. Conversely, augmentation of miRNA-124 restored cognitive function after repeated TBI.[219]

A fascinating example of microRNA expression that impacts the CAP was reported, again, by Soreq and colleagues in 2017, when they described the role of miRNA-211 in epilepsy. Recall from chapter 2 that acetylcholine is a critical regulator of seizure potential, and withdrawal of it can lead to a heightened risk of seizure. miRNA-211 regulates the expression of the 7 subunit of the nAChR. The practical upshot of this is that miRNA-211 expression suppresses seizures. Conversely, blocking of the miRNA-211 leads to enhanced seizure risk caused by dysfunctional acetylcholine activity (and dysregulated calcium flow).[220] VNS upregulates miRNA-211 expression and reduces seizure risk.

In 2019, Sanders and colleagues published a paper investigating the underlying mechanisms behind the cognition-enhancing effects of VNS. (In the authors' words, "Vagus nerve stimulation (VNS) has been shown to facilitate plasticity and memory in animal models and humans.") The results from their series of animal studies confirmed that VNS modulates gene expression in multiple categories, including epigenetic regulators (e.g., DNMTs and histone methylation/demethylation proteins).[221]

In their study, the potency of the VNS effect was so strong that protein expression levels of epigenetic regulators were so different between the sham and VNS groups that the brain tissue could be clearly distinguished by these levels alone. (Recall that the hippocampus is where learning and memory formation occurs.)

LONGEVITY AND VNS

The field of antiaging medicine is both nascent and ancient. In every culture since before the dawn of history, mankind has sought potions, spells, and talismans to provide eternal youth. The molecular and cellular processes that drive aging, however, have only recently begun to relinquish their secrets. As such, the migration of the field from the stuff of theology and mysticism into the light of science has only recently occurred. In 2013, Lopez-Otin and colleagues laid out the lines of scientific investigation that were most likely to decode the phenomenon of aging. Among other factors (including telomere length, cellular senescence, stem cell depletion, dysregulated nutrient sensing, and altered intercellular communication), Lopez-Otin suggested that aging could be explained through epigenetic modifications, instability within the genome and the proteome, and a degradation of mitochondrial health. The remainder of this section is focused on what that looks like and how to modulate it.[222]

The fundamental purpose of epigenetic mechanisms is to provide the means to adjust protein expression to meet demands encountered throughout life. Demands for the full complement of genes in a species' genome rapidly declines with development as cellular specialization occurs so that by birth, nearly all the cells (other than stem cells) have up to 60 to 80 percent of their genes sequestered away. As we age, however, genes that were previously sequestered efficiently become "loose," and the marks on the DNA and histones that repressed protein expression become altered. Sometimes this change is the result of a transient need to access an otherwise sequestered gene, but other times it is a function of ROS damage, toxins, radiation, or other chemical modifying agents. Because of these mechanisms, there appears to be an inexorable slide toward a loss of repression of protein expression. This is especially prominent at the ends of chromosomes (telomere-containing regions) and around the centromeres (which are typically H3K9me3 marked regions).[223] For those looking to slow aging processes, it was a natural question to ask whether there might be ways to inhibit that progression. Tantalizingly, the answer appears that it may be yes.

Most of the evidence for epigenetic changes that influence lifespan are, by necessity, the result of animal experiments (the invention of tools for studying many epigenetic marks are simply too recent (i.e., the past few years, to have gathered longevity results in most larger animal models). Still, we have intriguing data, such as the depletion of LSD-1 (lysine-specific demethylase), which is an H3K4 demethylase, has been reported to extend lifespan in some primitive species.[224] Remember that H3K4 methylation typically enhances protein expression, so removal of those marks suppresses protein expression, and this is associated with enhanced lifespan.

Conversely, methylation of H3K27 has repressive effects on protein expression. It is not surprising, therefore, that aging is associated with reductions in H3K27me3, leading to more protein expression. So, H3K27me3 reduces protein expression, and aging is associated with a loss of these marks. With this in mind, Anne Brunet and colleagues investigated an H3K27me3 demethylase, UTX-1, which would remove these marks and enhance aging. What they found was, mutation or deletion of the UTX-1 gene that disables the demethylase led to increases in H3K27me3, and it extended lifespan.[225]

Similarly, one of the earliest examples showing how altering histone methylase can affect lifespan is the mutation of COMPASS, which as discussed when H3K4 promotion was first described. In a primitive animal called *C. elegans* (a nematode, which is a very simple worm-like creature), disabling COMPASS leads to a longer lifespan (by some measures, double!) Fascinatingly, if an animal with this mutation is mated with one that has a normal COMPASS gene, the offspring have one functional and one nonfunctional COMPASS gene, but the offspring (and their progeny for at least one more generation) still experience COMPASS suppression and extended lifespan.[226]

These findings suggest two things: first, that suppressing protein expression can be lifespan enhancing, and second, that some life extending epigenetic changes can be inherited. Let's tackle these topics in the same order.

CALORIC RESTRICTION AND LIFESPAN

It has long been known that caloric restriction can lead to an extended lifespan. One of the presumed mechanisms for this longevity effect is the inhibition of protein expression that comes from a lack of nutrients. In addition, or more specifically, evidence suggests that nutrient deficiency leads to autophagy, which is at the heart of the life-extending benefits of near starvation (or at least intermittent fasting).[227] How does that work, you ask?

Autophagy is an internal cellular process that involves the formation of a membrane enclosed region, the *autophagosome*, that contains excess and/or unnecessary contents within its volume. The bubble of superfluous material is then merged with a lysosome (a similar bubble filled with enzymes and other caustic materials) to tear apart (i.e., lyse, and recycle the contents of the autophagosome). Autophagy is most prominently observed during periods when access to outside nutrients is limited, so the cell needs to rely on recycling to gain access to the molecules it needs.[228]

At the molecular level, caloric restriction activates autophagy by the suppression of mTOR (mammalian target of rapamycin–a protein complex that regulates multiple pathways, including proliferation and apoptosis). In short, mTOR is a nutrient sensor, and when nutrients are not plentiful (e.g., calorie restriction), mTOR is deactivated and autophagy is engaged. This means that mTOR activity and autophagy are opposing modes of cellular function.[229]

In 2019, Antonis Kirmizis and colleagues published a broad survey paper describing the interplay of diet, histone modification, and longevity, and, as the title of their paper (*Histone Modifications as an Intersection Between Diet and Longevity*), the effects of diet on longevity appear to correlate with changes in histone methylation, and these pathways are tied to specific biochemical pathways tightly associated with inflammation. In their words:

> [H]istone modifications act as an intermediate between diet and longevity. Calorie restriction (CR), high fat (HF), low protein (LP), single nutrient (SN) conditions are sensed by the cell through signaling pathways like TOR, Ras, AMPK or PI3K/AKT, promoting changes on the epigenome ... [that] have been consistently linked to a particular lifespan effect and are shown within the respective cell nucleus.[230]

The dynamics of the mTOR pathway have been studied, and not surprisingly, it is a prime example of what Lopez-Otin referred to as dysregulated nutrient sensing in aging. That is, with advancing age, there is a gradual loss of mechanisms that moderate mTOR activity, and it shifts into a permanently active state. In fact, RNA sequencing of centenarians, their spouses, and their children has revealed that genes coding for proteins that make up the autophagosome (e.g., ATGs) are more readily expressed (meaning mTOR is still being suppressed) in those who reach 100 years of age as compared with their contemporaries who did not.[231]

Consistent with this finding, another gene known as RPTOR (regulatory associated protein of the mTOR complex) was suppressed in those who made it a century.[232] RPTOR is expressed and activated to support mTOR activity by increased amino acid levels and through glucose stimulated insulin receptor activity. Reduced expression of RPTOR is, therefore, associated with a low level of nutrition.

Let's take a step back for a moment to get our bearings. How should we process this information that near starvation dieting and intermittent fasting is actually good for having our lifespans extended (and it reduces cancer risks, the probability of cardiovascular disease, neurodegenerative disorders, and obviously lowers the chances of obesity-related metabolic disease)? Why is it that being smart enough, or strong enough, to get more food is actually a bad thing for our bodies?

A helpful perspective is to realize that most of life on the planet actually struggles to find sufficient food to survive. Many of the rest gorge themselves during brief periods of plenty (like bears during salmon spawning periods) in advance of a long winter of fasting through hibernation. This was the life our human ancestors lived for millennia, and really up until the last eighty years. (And as chapter 3 explained, widespread use of refrigeration, the chemistry of food preservatives, population-scale food production, and efficient food transportation and logistics made food available to the point that metabolic syndrome is now a pandemic-scale problem, and our bodies have not evolved to handle the overnutrition problem.) Our bodies, and those of our ancestors, spanning hundreds of millions of years, evolved to function most efficiently under conditions of food scarcity. We are driven to eat, even crave, foods with exceptionally high levels of nutrients; even those who appear most strong and fit are actually chronically living in a state of overnutrition. While weight loss in the elderly, especially unexpected or unintentional weight loss, can be a concern, getting thin prior to entering older age isn't just good for your heart and your joints, it enables the mTOR pathway to be switched off and for autophagy to remain active for longer.

Digging into the science, the deactivation of mTOR that takes place through caloric restriction occurs through multiple pathways, involving modulation of insulin signaling (IIS, associated with food intake), mitochondrial energy output (AMPK), and deacetylation and autophagy activation by sirtuin proteins (SIRT).[233] To be more specific about AMPK, during periods of nutrient scarcity, levels of AMP and ADP (the depleted batteries for the cellular tools) rise as mitochondria have a reduced ability to regenerate ATP. This leads to the activation of AMP-activated protein kinase (AMPK), which is a cellular energy sensing enzyme that detects the relative levels of AMP/ADP to ATP that blocks mTOR activity. AMPK actually promotes the proliferation of new mitochondria and increases activity of a protein, ULK1, which promotes autophagy.[234]

So, we have discussed some of the mechanisms by which caloric restriction affects longevity, many of which relate to either the clearing out of excessive amounts of cellular debris (autophagy) or the repression of protein expression (epigenetic marking). This leads to the second question that was asked above: Are these marks inherited, and if so, do these epigenetic changes have positive or negative effects on the lifespans of progeny?

ALTERED GENE EXPRESSION AND LIFESPAN

Studies in animals have shown that thousands of genes have altered expression levels associated with calorie restriction. Many of clusters of these changes are associated with more than a dozen functions relating to metabolism, from glucose metabolism (insulin signaling) to mitochondrial function. Interestingly, the changes in protein expression levels are correlated with modulation of DNMTs (the methyltransferases that methylate DNA). Even short-term caloric restriction leads to alterations in the DNA methylation of genes for metabolism and inflammatory cytokines (e.g., TNF-α), delays aging, and reduces the risk of cancer.[235] In some cases, this modulation leads to a maintenance of DNA methylation that is otherwise slowly being lost in the aging animals. Conversely, inhibition of DNMTs responsible for methylation of autophagy-associated proteins restores more youthful autophagy stimulation.[236]

Inhibition of protein translation by non-coding RNA has a role in autophagy, as well.[237] Specifically, low nutrient and energy conditions are associated with modulation in the levels of hundreds of miRNAs that target aspects of the mTOR pathway and autophagy. Although these studies are typically carried out in cultured cell lines, in vitro, the deprivation of oxygen, glucose, and other nutrients activate miRNAs like miRNA-211 that promote autophagy through targeting mTOR, RPTOR, and aspects of the insulin pathway.

Predictably, there are miRNAs that work the other side of the equation (i.e., inhibiting autophagy) by targeting sirtuin proteins, ULK1, and a host of autophagosomal proteins. Two such miRNAs are miRNA-30A and miRNA-34A.[238]

The microRNAs are often associated with vagus nerve stimulation, including miRNA-155 and miRNA-210. Both have bidirectional influences on autophagy *in vitro*. miRNA-210, which reportedly mediates the positive effects of vagus nerve stimulation in epilepsy, seems to enhance autophagy in some cases, but inhibits it in others.[239] Is there an anti-autophagy function of these miRNAs during severe inflammation, refocusing stressed cells toward other activities rather than autophagy? Much research still needs to be done to answer important questions about VNS, ncRNA, and longevity.

CAN WE INHERIT LONGEVITY?

All of this leads to the final (compound) question of the chapter, which is: Can epigenetic changes related to longevity and/or autophagy be transmitted to subsequent generations, and if so, by what mechanism does this inheritance occur?

Observations made for at least the past 100 years suggest the answer to the first part should be yes. In 1918, forty-two years after inventing the telephone, Alexander Graham Bell wrote a paper in which he asserted that children born to young mothers have longer lifespans than children born to older mothers. This effect is now, somewhat unfairly, referred to as the Lansing Effect, named for Albert Lansing who wrote about it in 1947, nearly thirty years after Bell's original paper. While the fundamental assertion has been challenged by some, the majority of subsequent research, across species from fruit flies to humans, has been supportive. Given the combination of age-related methylation state changes that have been observed in the egg cells of older animals, and the potential for inheritance of these marks, it is not unreasonable to suggest that Bell's observation may be accurate, and that epigenetic inheritance leads to changes in lifespan (positive or negative).[240]

As discussed previously, studies from the Netherlands have shown that starvation of the mother during pregnancy has negative mental health outcomes for the child. Further investigation has shown that lifespans among the grandchildren are also negatively impacted. In contrast to these studies in which mothers were suffering with malnutrition *during* pregnancy, a study of the effects of childhood starvation on the health of subsequent generations was conducted in Sweden by Bygren and colleagues, looking at the progeny of those who suffered through a failed harvest in the mid-1800s.[241] What their work revealed was that childhood hunger positively affects health and lifespan, and that these effects extend multigenerationally, in what can be a sex-dependent manner.

More specifically, the Bygren data showed that lack of food among prepubescent boys afforded extended lifespan in the grandchildren (a transgenerational effect). Lack of food for grandfathers during their formative years afforded their grandsons with an average lifespan six years longer than among those who experienced no periods of starvation (it has been reported that correcting for socioeconomic factors, the lifespan enhancement was actually an astounding thirty-two years!) Coupled with these lifespan-extending benefits were fewer metabolic syndrome complications (CVD and diabetes). Looking at larger populations, subsequent work in Sweden has confirmed these benefits with respect to cancer and "all-cause" mortality. These benefits appear to be sex-biased in that childhood malnutrition among females led to a higher incidence of death from CVD mortality and no benefits with respect to cancer.

The second part of the compound question above asks what mechanism or mechanisms are involved with this inheritance of enhanced or inhibited longevity and autophagy. While inheritance of select DNA methylation sites appears to survive demethylation processes that accompany the post-fertilization cleansing of the germline genome, as Li-Fang Hu writes, "The impact of DNA methylation on autophagy may be tissue- or cell-specific," but "the study on autophagy regulation by DNA methylation is still in its infancy."[242]

Compared with DNA methylation, there is modestly better knowledge of how histone modification regulates autophagy, and how these modifications may be inherited. For example, one pathway to the activation of autophagy involves the acetylation of H4K16 by KAT8 (a histone acetyltransferase, or HAT), which initiates autophagy gene transcription, and increases with the expression of the deacetylase, SIRT1. The expression of KAT8 can be maternally inherited, and its effects on increased lifespan through H4K16 acetylation appears to be maintained from the egg-sourced genetic material, through fertilization in mouse models.[243]

Perhaps most influential on the inheritance of longevity-influencing gene expression, however, including predisposition to autophagy, are microRNAs. More specifically, miRNA-71 (along with miRNA-238 and miRNA-246) has been identified as enhancing longevity, while miRNA-34 and miRNA-239 appear to inhibit it.[244] Disabling mutations of miRNA-34 extend lifespan through an autophagy-dependent pathway, and miRNA-239 loss-of-function extends the lifespan through an insulin signaling/AMPK pathway. Evidence for these gene-silencing RNAs, including starvation-induced miRNAs (and associated increased lifespan), being inherited through at least three generations has been shown in multiple animal models. How does this occur?

Recall that microRNA bind to the messenger RNA and gum up the protein manufacturing processes by inhibiting the ribosome and/or causing the messenger RNA template to be digested away. Unlike methylation of DNA or histones (or other modifications of the latter), miRNA function outside of the nucleus from DNA that is replicated and requires subsequent processing to restore the epigenetic marks. After initial transcription and sequence modification steps, the argonaute protein coupled with the miRNA exists in the cytosol, so half of the miRNAs pass to the daughter cell and half remain with the parent cell. During periods of significant cell division, such germline cell development, the daughter cells have mechanisms in place to ensure that any deficit of the proteins in the cell that occur as a result of cell division is rectified. Similar mechanisms are present for the maintenance of miRNA levels as well, provided that the genes involved were expressed in the germline. [245] Genes directed to nutrition are expressed in the germline, and they have been the ones identified as being targeted by the miRNAs that are inherited and have their levels maintained through multiple generations.

In conclusion, while we have no control over our mothers' ages when they gave birth to us, caloric restriction and intermittent fasting are actions we can take to enhance our lifespans.

Together with the timing of when we choose to have our future children (or encourage our own children to procreate), dietary inducement or other means of triggering autophagy may impart longevity to our descendants.

ENDNOTES

1 W. Karczewski and J. G. Widdicombe, "The Role of the Vagus Nerves in the Respiratory and Circulatory Reactions to Anaphylaxis in Rabbits," *The Journal of Physiology* 201, no. 2 (1969): 293–304.

2 Elmin Steyn, Mohamed Zunaid, and Carla Husselman, "Non-invasive Vagus Nerve Stimulation for the Treatment of Acute Asthma Exacerbations—Results from an Initial Case Series," *International Journal of Emergency Medicine* 6, no. 1 (2013): 1–3.

3 Lyudmila V. Borovikova, et al.,"Vagus Nerve Stimulation Attenuates the Systemic Inflammatory Response to Endotoxin," *Nature* 405, no. 6785 (2000): 458–462.

4 Ulf Andersson and Kevin J. Tracey, "Reflex Principles of Immunological Homeostasis," *Annual Review of Immunology* 30 (2012): 313–335.

5 Javier Egea, et al., "Anti-Inflammatory Role of Microglial Alpha7 nAChRs and Its Role in Neuroprotection," *Biochemical Pharmacology* 97, no. 4 (2015): 463–472.

6 Galyna Gergalova, et al., "Mitochondria Express A7 Nicotinic Acetylcholine Receptors to Regulate Ca2+ Accumulation and Cytochrome C Release: Study on Isolated Mitochondria," *PloS One* 7, no. 2 (2012): e31361.

7 Ben Lu, et al., "α7 Nicotinic Acetylcholine Receptor Signaling Inhibits Inflammasome Activation by Preventing Mitochondrial DNA Release," *Molecular Medicine* 20 (2014): 350–358.

8 Francoise Alliot, Isabelle Godin, and Bernard Pessac, "Microglia Derive from Progenitors, Originating from the Yolk Sac, and Which Proliferate in the Brain," *Developmental Brain Research* 117, no. 2 (1999): 145–152.

9 Jeffrey L. Frost and Dorothy P. Schafer, "Microglia: Architects of the Developing Nervous System," *Trends in Cell Biology* 26, no. 8 (2016):

587–597; Akiko Miyamoto, "Microglia Contact Induces Synapse Formation in Developing Somatosensory Cortex," *Nature Communications* 7, no. 1 (2016): 12540; Kaoru Sato, "Effects of Microglia on Neurogenesis," *Glia* 63, no. 8 (2015): 1394–1405; Joana R. Guedes, Pedro A. Ferreira, Jéssica M. Costa, Ana L. Cardoso, and João Peça, "Microglia-Dependent Remodeling of Neuronal Circuits," *Journal of Neurochemistry* 163, no. 2 (2022): 74–93.

10 Rosa C. Paolicelli and Cornelius T. Gross, "Microglia in Development: Linking Brain Wiring to Brain Environment," *Neuron Glia Biology* 7, no. 1 (2011): 77–83.

11 Georgia Gunner Faust and Dorothy P. Schafer, "Mechanisms Governing Activity-Dependent Synaptic Pruning in the Developing Mammalian CNS," *Nature Reviews Neuroscience* 22, no. 11 (2021): 657–673.

12 Yuwen Wu, Lasse Dissing-Olesen, Brian A. MacVicar, and Beth Stevens, "Microglia: Dynamic Mediators of Synapse Development and Plasticity," *Trends in Immunology* 36, no. 10 (2015): 605–613; Roger A. Nicoll, "A Brief History of Long-Term Potentiation," *Neuron* 93, no. 2 (2017): 281–290.

13 Yuki Hattori, "The Microglia-Blood Vessel Interactions in the Developing Brain," *Neuroscience Research* (2022); David A. Menassa and Diego Gomez-Nicola, "Microglial Dynamics during Human Brain Development," *Frontiers in Immunology* 9 (2018): 1014.

14 Akio Suzumura, "Neuron-Microglia Interaction in Neuroinflammation," *Current Protein and Peptide Science* 14, no. 1 (2013): 16–20.

15 Mar Márquez-Ropero, Eva Benito, Ainhoa Plaza-Zabala, and Amanda Sierra, "Microglial Corpse Clearance: Lessons from Macrophages," *Frontiers in Immunology* 11 (2020): 506.

16 Meiyan Wang, Lei Zhang, and Fred H. Gage, "Microglia, Complement and Schizophrenia," *Nature Neuroscience* 22, no. 3 (2019): 333–334; Ryuta Koyama, and Yuji Ikegaya, "Microglia in the Pathogenesis of Autism Spectrum Disorders," *Neuroscience Research* 100 (2015): 1–5.

17 Christine T. Ekdahl, "Microglial Activation–Tuning and Pruning Adult Neurogenesis," *Frontiers in Pharmacology* 3 (2012): 41.

18 Gang Chen, et al., "Microglia in Pahin: Detrimental and Protective Roles in Pathogenesis and Resolution of Pain," *Neuron* 100, no. 6 (2018): 1292-1311.; Raz Yirmiya, Neta Rimmerman, and Ronen Reshef,

"Depression as a Microglial Disease," *Trends in Neurosciences* 38, no. 10 (2015): 637–658; Haixia Wang, et al., "Microglia in Depression: An Overview of Microglia in the Pathogenesis and Treatment of Depression," *Journal of Neuroinflammation* 19, no. 1 (2022): 132; Karol Ramirez, Jaime Fornaguera-Trías, and John F. Sheridan, "Stress-Induced Microglia Activation and Monocyte Trafficking to the Brain Underlie the Development of Anxiety and Depression," *Inflammation-Associated Depression: Evidence, Mechanisms, and Implications* (2017): 155–172; Michael R. Irwin, "Sleep and inflammation: Partners in Sickness and in Health," *Nature Reviews Immunology* 19, no. 11 (2019): 702–715; Xiang Zhang, et al.,"Activated Brain Mast Cells Contribute to Postoperative Cognitive Dysfunction by Evoking Microglia Activation and Neuronal Apoptosis," *Journal of Neuroinflammation* 13, no. 1 (2016): 1–15; Xiaofeng Zhao, et al., "Noninflammatory Changes of Microglia are Sufficient to Cause Epilepsy," *Cell Reports* 22, no. 8 (2018): 2080–2093; Wolfgang J. Streit, Kelly R. Miller, Kryslaine O. Lopes, and Emalick Njie, "Microglial Degeneration in the Aging Brain–Bad News for Neurons," *Frontiers in Bioscience* 13 (2008): 3423–3438.

19   Lil Qui, et al., "Macrophages at the Crossroad of Meta-Inflammation and Inflammaging," *Genes* 13, no. 11 (2022): 2074.

20   Cynthia M. Solek, et al., "Maternal Immune Activation in Neurodevelopmental Disorders," *Developmental Dynamics* 247, no. 4 (2018): 588–619; Irene Knuesel, et al.,"Maternal Immune Activation and Abnormal Brain Development Across CNS Disorders," *Nature Reviews Neurology* 10, no. 11 (2014): 643–660; Marianela E. Traetta and Marie-Ève Tremblay, "Prenatal Inflammation Shapes Microglial Immune Response into Adulthood," *Trends in Immunology* (2022); Kana Ozaki, et al., "Maternal Immune Activation Induces Sustained Changes in Fetal Microglia Motility," *Scientific Reports* 10, no. 1 (2020): 21378.

21   Marianela E. Traetta and Marie-Ève Tremblay, "Prenatal Inflammation Shapes Microglial Immune Response into Adulthood," *Trends in Immunology* (2022); Sophia M. Loewen, et al., "The Outcomes of Maternal Immune Activation Induced with the Viral Mimetic Poly I: C on Microglia in Exposed Rodent Offspring," *Developmental Neuroscience* (2023); Maude Bordeleau, Lourdes Fernandez de Cossio, M. Mallar Chakravarty, and Marie-Ève Tremblay, "From Maternal Diet to Neurodevelopmental Disorders: A Story of Neuroinflammation,"

Frontiers in Cellular Neuroscience 14 (2021): 612705; Tara C.Delorme, William Ozell-Landry, Nicolas Cermakian, and Lalit K. Srivastava, "Behavioral and Cellular Responses to Circadian Disruption and Prenatal Immune Activation in Mice," *Scientific Reports* 13, no. 1 (2023): 7791; Marek Kubicki, Robert W. McCarley, and Martha E. Shenton, "Evidence for White Matter Abnormalities in Schizophrenia," *Current Opinion in Psychiatry* 18, no. 2 (2005): 121.

22   Alan S. Brown, "Epidemiologic Studies of Exposure to Prenatal Infection and Risk of Schizophrenia and Autism," *Developmental Neurobiology* 72, no. 10 (2012): 1272–1276; Alan S. Brown and Elena J. Derkits, "Prenatal Infection and Schizophrenia: A Review of Epidemiologic and Translational Studies," *American Journal of Psychiatry* 167, no. 3 (2010): 261–280; Sarah Canetta, et al.,"Elevated Maternal C-Reactive Protein and Increased Risk of Schizophrenia in a National Birth Cohort," *American Journal of Psychiatry* 171, no. 9 (2014): 960–968.

23   Elisa Guma, et al., "Differential Effects of Early or Late Exposure to Prenatal Maternal Immune Activation on Mouse Embryonic Neurodevelopment," *Proceedings of the National Academy of Sciences* 119, no. 12 (2022): e2114545119.

24   Hjördis Ó. Atladóttir, et al., "Maternal Infection Requiring Hospitalization during Pregnancy and Autism Spectrum Disorders," *Journal of Autism and Developmental Disorders* 40 (2010): 1423–1430; Manuel F. López-Aranda, et al., "Postnatal Immune Activation Causes Social Deficits in a Mouse Model of Tuberous Sclerosis: Role of Microglia and Clinical Implications," *Science Advances* 7, no. 38 (2021): eabf2073.

25   Parboosing, Raveen, Yuanyuan Bao, Ling Shen, Catherine A. Schaefer, and Alan S. Brown, "Gestational Influenza and Bipolar Disorder in Adult Offspring," *JAMA Psychiatry* 70, no. 7 (2013): 677–685.

26   Timothy C. Nielsen, et al., "Association of Maternal Autoimmune Disease with Attention-Deficit/Hyperactivity Disorder in Children," *JAMA Pediatrics* 175, no. 3 (2021): e205487; Johanne T. Instanes, et al., "Attention-Deficit/Hyperactivity Disorder in Offspring of Mothers with Inflammatory and Immune System Diseases," *Biological Psychiatry* 81, no. 5 (2017): 452–459.

27   Geoffrey A. Dunn, Joel T. Nigg, and Elinor L. Sullivan, "Neuroinflam-mation as a Risk Factor for Attention Deficit Hyperactivity Disorder," *Pharmacology Biochemistry and Behavior* 182 (2019): 22–34.

28 Paul H. Patterson, "Maternal Infection and Immune Involvement in Autism," *Trends in Molecular Medicine* 17, no. 7 (2011): 389–394.

29 Megumi Andoh, Yuji Ikegaya, and Ryuta Koyama, "Microglia as Possible Therapeutic Targets for Autism Spectrum Disorders," *Progress in Molecular Biology and Translational Science* 167 (2019): 223–245.

30 Marilynn Marchione, "Chinese Researcher Claims First Gene-Edited Babies," *AP News*, November 16, 2018, https://apnews.com/article/ap -top-news-international-news-ca-state-wire-genetic-frontiers-health -4997bb7aa36c45449b488e19ac83e86d; Antonio Regalado, "Chinese Scientists Are Creating CRISPR Babies," *MIT Technology Review*, November 25, 2018, https://www.technologyreview.com/2018/11/25 /138962/exclusive-chinese-scientists-are-creating-crispr-babies.

31 Miou Zhou, et al., "CCR5 is a Suppressor for Cortical Plasticity and Hippocampal Learning and Memory," *Elife* 5 (2016): e20985.

32 Tilendra Choudhary, et al., "Effect of Transcutaneous Cervical Vagus Nerve Stimulation on Declarative and Working Memory in Patients with Posttraumatic Stress Disorder (PTSD): A Pilot Study," *Journal of Affective Disorders* 339 (2023): 418–425.

33 Véronique Desbeaumes Jodoin, et al., "Long-Term Sustained Cognitive Benefits of Vagus Nerve Stimulation in Refractory Depression," *The Journal of ECT* 34, no. 4 (2018): 283–290.

34 Chun-Hong Liu, et al., "Neural Networks and the Anti-Inflammatory Effect of Transcutaneous Auricular Vagus Nerve Stimulation in Depression," *Journal of Neuroinflammation* 17, no. 1 (2020): 1–11.

35 Andy McKinley McIntire, Chuck Goodyear, John P. McIntire, and Rebecca D. Brown, "Cervical Transcutaneous Vagal Nerve Stimulation (Ctvns) Improves Human Cognitive Performance under Sleep Deprivation Stress," *Communications Biology* 4, no. 1 (2021): 634; Toshiya Miyatsu, et al., "Transcutaneous Cervical Vagus Nerve Stimulation Enhances Second-Language Vocabulary Acquisition While Simultaneously Mitigating Fatigue and Promoting Focus (P2-12.002)," *Neurology* 100 (2023); Lindsey McIntire, Andy McKinley, and Melissa Key, "Cervical Transcutaneous Vagal Nerve Stimulation to Improve Mission Qualification Training for an AFSOC Full Motion Video/Geospatial Analysis Squadron," *Brain Stimulation: Basic, Translational, and Clinical Research in Neuromodulation* 16, no. 1 (2023): 229.

36 Ann Mertens, et al., "The Potential of Invasive and Non-Invasive Vagus Nerve Stimulation to Improve Verbal Memory Performance in Epilepsy Patients," *Scientific Reports* 12, no. 1 (2022): 1984.

37 National Institute of Mental Health, "Major Depression," NIMH, Last updated July 2023, https://www.nimh.nih.gov/health/statistics /major-depression; National Institute of Mental Health, "Any Anxiety Disorder," NIMH, Accessed October 16, 2023, https://www.nimh.nih.gov /health/statistics/any-anxiety-disorder#part_2576; National institute of Mental Health, "Post-Traumatic Stress Disorder (PTSD)," NIMH, Accessed October 18, 2023, https://www.nimh.nih.gov/health/statistics/post -traumatic-stress-disorder-ptsd.

38 Shai Mulinari, "Monoamine Theories of Depression: Historical Impact on Biomedical Research," *Journal of the History of the Neurosciences* 21, no. 4 (2012): 366–392.

39 Irvine H. Page, "Serotonin," *Scientific American* 197, no. 6 (1957): 52–57; Mikwang Kwon, Murat Altin, Hector Duenas, and Levent Alev, "The Role of Descending Inhibitory Pathways on Chronic Pain Modulation and Clinical Implications," *Pain Practice* 14, no. 7 (2014): 656-667.

40 John Ioannidis, "Effectiveness of Antidepressants: An Evidence Myth Constructed from a Thousand Randomized Trials?" *Philosophy, Ethics, and Humanities in Medicine* 3, no. 1 (2008): 1–9; John Walkup and Michael Labellarte, "Complications of SSRI Treatment," *Journal of Child and Adolescent Psychopharmacology* 11, no. 1 (2001): 1–4.

41 Nicole Lichtblau, et al., "Cytokines as Biomarkers in Depressive Disorder: Current Standing and Prospects," *International Review of Psychiatry* 25, no. 5 (2013): 592–603.

42 C. R. MacKenzie, K. Heseler, A. Muller, and Walter Daubener, "Role of Indoleamine 2, 3-Dioxygenase in Antimicrobial Defence and Immuno-Regulation: Tryptophan Depletion versus Production of Toxic Kynurenines," *Current Drug Metabolism* 8, no. 3 (2007): 237–244; Aye Mu Myint and Yong Ku Kim, "Cytokine–Serotonin Interaction through IDO: A Neurodegeneration Hypothesis of Depression," *Medical Hypotheses* 61, no. 5–6 (2003): 519–525.

43 M. Elizabeth Sublette, et al., "Plasma Kynurenine Levels Are Elevated in Suicide Attempters with Major Depressive Disorder," *Brain, Behavior, and Immunity* 25, no. 6 (2011): 1272–1278; Kamiyu Ogyu, et al., "Kynurenine Pathway in Depression: A Systematic Review and

Meta-Analysis," *Neuroscience & Biobehavioral Reviews* 90 (2018): 16–25; Luca Sforzini, Maria Antonietta Nettis, Valeria Mondelli, and Carmine Maria Pariante, "Inflammation in Cancer and Depression: A Starring Role for the Kynurenine Pathway," *Psychopharmacology* 236 (2019): 2997–3011; Simon P. Jones, et al., "Expression of the Kynurenine Pathway in Human Peripheral Blood Mononuclear Cells: Implications for Inflammatory and Neurodegenerative Disease," *PloS One* 10, no. 6 (2015): e0131389; Caroline M. Forrest, et al., "Purine, Kynurenine, Neopterin, and Lipid Peroxidation Levels in Inflammatory Bowel Disease," *Journal of Biomedical Science* 9, no. 5 (2002): 436–442; Roland Baumgartner, Maria J. Forteza, and Daniel F. J. Ketelhuth, "The Interplay Between Cytokines and the Kynurenine Pathway in Inflammation and Atherosclerosis," *Cytokine* 122 (2019): 154148.

44 Chieh-Hsin Lee and Fabrizio Giuliani, "The Role of Inflammation in Depression and Fatigue," *Frontiers in Immunology* 10 (2019): 1696; G. Anderson and Michael Maes, "Mitochondria and Immunity in Chronic Fatigue Syndrome," *Progress in Neuro-Psychopharmacology and Biological Psychiatry* 103 (2020): 109976.

45 Sandra Malynn, Antonio Campos-Torres, Paul Moynagh, and Jana Haase, "The Pro-Inflammatory Cytokine TNF-A Regulates the Activity and Expression of the Serotonin Transporter (SERT) in Astrocytes," *Neurochemical Research* 38 (2013): 694–704.

46 Xiao-Xia Dong, Yan Wang, and Zheng-Hong Qin, "Molecular Mechanisms of Excitotoxicity and their Relevance to Pathogenesis of Neurodegenerative Diseases," *Acta Pharmacologica Sinica* 30, no. 4 (2009): 379–387.

47 Jessica Tarn, Sarah Legg, Sheryl Mitchell, Bruce Simon, and Wan-Fai Ng, "The Effects of Noninvasive Vagus Nerve Stimulation on Fatigue and Immune Responses in Patients with Primary Sjögren's Syndrome," *Neuromodulation: Technology at the Neural Interface* 22, no. 5 (2019): 580–585; Jessica Tarn, et al., "The Effects of Noninvasive Vagus Nerve Stimulation on Fatigue in Participants with Primary Sjögren's Syndrome," *Neuromodulation: Technology at the Neural Interface* 26, no. 3 (2023): 681–689.

48 Dario Acuna-Castroviejo, Germaine Escames, Maria I. Rodriguez, and Luis C. Lopez, "Melatonin Role in the Mitochondrial Function," *Frontiers in Bioscience-Landmark* 12, no. 3 (2007): 947–963.

49   Russel J. Reiter, et al., "Melatonin: A Mitochondrial Resident with a Diverse Skill Set," *Life Sciences* 301 (2022): 120612.

50   Joel S. Riley and Stephen W. G. Tait, "Mitochondrial DNA in Inflammation and Immunity," *EMBO Reports* 21, no. 4 (2020): e49799; Jeonghan Kim, Ho-Shik Kim, and Jay H. Chung, "Molecular Mechanisms of Mitochondrial DNA Release and Activation of the cGAS-STING Sathway," *Experimental & Molecular Medicine* 55, no. 3 (2023): 510–519.

51   N. Tabassum, et al., "A Review on the Possible Leakage of Electrons through the Electron Transport Chain within Mitochondria," *Life Science* 6 (2020): 105–113; Alexander L. Chernorudskiy and Ester Zito, "Regulation of Calcium Homeostasis by ER Redox: A Close-Up of the ER/Mitochondria Connection," *Journal of Molecular Biology* 429, no. 5 (2017): 620–632.

52   P. A. Parone, D. James, and J. C. Martinou, "Mitochondria: Regulating the Inevitable," *Biochimie* 84, no. 2-3 (2002): 105–111.

53   Santhosh Satapati, et al., "Mitochondrial Metabolism Mediates Oxidative Stress and Inflammation in Fatty Liver," *The Journal of Clinical Investigation* 125, no. 12 (2015): 4447–4462.

54   Ben Lu, et al., "α7 Nicotinic Acetylcholine Receptor Signaling Inhibits Inflammasome Activation by Preventing Mitochondrial DNA Release," *Molecular Medicine* 20 (2014): 350–358.

55   Paul S. Brookes, et al., "Calcium, ATP, and ROS: A Mitochondrial Love-Hate Triangle," *American Journal of Physiology-Cell Physiology* (2004); György Hajnóczky, et al., "Mitochondrial Calcium Signaling and Cell Death: Approaches for Assessing the Role of Mitochondrial Ca2+ Uptake in Apoptosis," *Cell Calcium* 40, no. 5-6 (2006): 553–560; Galyna Gergalova, et al., "Mitochondria Express A7 Nicotinic Acetylcholine Receptors to Regulate Ca2+ Accumulation and Cytochrome C Release: Study on Isolated Mitochondria," *PloS One* 7, no. 2 (2012): e31361.

56   Katie Tolkien, Steven Bradburn, and Chris Murgatroyd, "An Anti-Inflammatory Diet as a Potential Intervention for Depressive Disorders: A Systematic Review and Meta-Analysis," (2018).

57   Ole Köhler-Forsberg, et al., "Efficacy of Anti-Inflammatory Treatment on Major Depressive Disorder or Depressive Symptoms: Meta-Analysis of Clinical Trials," *Acta Psychiatrica Scandinavica* 139, no. 5 (2019): 404-419; Norbert Müller, "COX-2 Inhibitors, Aspirin, and Other

Potential Anti-Inflammatory Treatments for Psychiatric Disorders,"
Frontiers in Psychiatry 10 (2019): 375.

58   Scott M. Berry, et al., "A Patient-Level Meta-Analysis of Studies
Evaluating Vagus Nerve Stimulation Therapy for Treatment-Resistant
Depression," *Medical Devices: Evidence and Research* (2013): 17–35.

59   Ying-Hao Ho, et al., "Peripheral Inflammation Increases Seizure
Susceptibility via the Induction of Neuroinflammation and Oxidative
Stress in the Hippocampus," *Journal of Biomedical Science* 22, no. 1
(2015): 1–14.

60   Jennifer C. Felger and Michael T. Treadway, "Inflammation
Effects on Motivation and Motor Activity: Role of Dopamine,"
Neuropsychopharmacology 42, no. 1 (2017): 216–241; Felix-Martin Werner
and Rafael Coveñas, "Classical Neurotransmitters and Neuropeptides
Involved in Generalized Epilepsy in a Multi-Neurotransmitter System:
How to Improve the Antiepileptic Effect?" *Epilepsy & Behavior* 71
(2017): 124–129; Shah Nigar, et al., "Molecular Insights into the Role of
Inflammation and Oxidative Stress in Epilepsy," *Journal of Advances
in Medical and Pharmaceutical Sciences* 10, no. 1 (2016): 1–9; Parizad
M. Bilimoria and Beth Stevens, "Microglia Function during Brain
Development: New Insights from Animal Models," *Brain Research* 1617
(2015): 7–17; Jennifer N. Pearson-Smith and Manisha Patel, "Metabolic
Dysfunction and Oxidative Stress in Epilepsy," *International Journal of
Molecular Sciences* 18, no. 11 (2017): 2365.

61   Tanya R. Victor and Stella E. Tsirka, "Microglial Contributions
to Aberrant Neurogenesis and Pathophysiology of Epilepsy,"
Neuroimmunology and Neuroinflammation 7 (2020): 234.

62   Gabriel Olmos and Jerònia Lladó, "Tumor Necrosis Factor Alpha:
A Link between Neuroinflammation and Excitotoxicity," *Mediators of
Inflammation* (2014).

63   Scott E. Krahl and Kevin B. Clark, "Vagus Nerve Stimulation
for Epilepsy: A Review of Central Mechanism," *Surgical Neurology
International* 3, no. 4 (2012): S255.

64   Enes Akyuz, et al., "Revisiting the Role of Neurotransmitters in
Epilepsy: An Updated Review," *Life Sciences* 265 (2021): 118826.

65   Jelena M. Pavlović, et al., "Burden of Migraine Related to Menses:
Results from the AMPP Study," *The Journal of Headache and Pain* 16,
no. 1 (2015): 1–11.

66   Michael L. Oshinsky and Sumittra Gomonchareonsiri, "Episodic Dural Stimulation in Awake Rats: A Model for Recurrent Headache," *Headache: The Journal of Head and Face Pain* 47, no. 7 (2007): 1026–1036.

67   Michael L. Oshinsky, et al., "Noninvasive Vagus Nerve Stimulation as Treatment for Trigeminal Allodynia," *Pain* 155, no. 5 (2014): 1037–1042.

68   Isabel Pavão Martins, "Crossed Aphasia during Migraine Aura: Transcallosal Spreading Depression?" *Journal of Neurology, Neurosurgery & Psychiatry* 78, no. 5 (2007): 544–545.

69   Cenk Ayata, et al., "Suppression of Cortical Spreading Depression in Migraine Prophylaxis," *Annals of Neurology: Official Journal of the American Neurological Association and the Child Neurology Society* 59, no. 4 (2006): 652–661.

70   Shih-Pin Chen and Cenk Ayatam, "Novel Therapeutic Targets Against Spreading Depression," *Headache: The Journal of Head and Face Pain* 57, no. 9 (2017): 1340–1358.

71   Kae M. Pusic, Aya D. Pusic, Jordan Kemme, and Richard P. Kraig, "Spreading Depression Requires Microglia and Is Decreased by Their M2a Polarization from Environmental Enrichment," *Glia* 62, no. 7 (2014): 1176–1194.

72   Shih-Pin Chen, et al., "Vagus Nerve Stimulation Inhibits Cortical Spreading Depression," *Pain* 157, no. 4 (2016): 797.

73   Elizabeth J. Bowen, et al., "Tumor Necrosis Factor—A Stimulation of Calcitonin Gene-Related Peptide Expression and Secretion from Rat Trigeminal Ganglion Neurons," *Journal of Neurochemistry* 96, no. 1 (2006): 65–77.

74   S. D. Brain, T. J. Williams, J. R. Tippins, H. R. Morris, and I. MacIntyre, "Calcitonin Gene-Related Peptide Is a Potent Vasodilator," *Nature* 313, no. 5997 (1985): 54–56.

75   Antoinette MaassenVanDenBrink, Joris Meijer, Carlos M. Villalón, and Michel D. Ferrari, "Wiping Out CGRP: Potential Cardiovascular Risks, " *Trends in Pharmacological Sciences* 37, no. 9 (2016): 779–788.

76   Jordan L. Hawkins, Lauren E. Cornelison, Brian A. Blankenship, and Paul L. Durham, "Vagus Nerve Stimulation Inhibits Trigeminal Nociception in a Rodent Model of Episodic Migraine," *Pain Reports* 2, no. 6 (2017); Romina Nassini, et al., "The 'Headache Tree' via Umbellulone and TRPA1 Activates the Trigeminovascular System," *Brain* 135, no. 2 (2012): 376–390; Lauren E. Cornelison, Jordan L. Hawkins, Sara E.

Woodman, and Paul L. Durham, "Noninvasive Vagus Nerve Stimulation and Morphine Transiently Inhibit Trigeminal Pain Signaling in a Chronic Headache Model," *Pain Reports* 5, no. 6 (2020).

77   Tzu-Ting Liu, et al., "Efficacy Profile of Noninvasive Vagus Nerve Stimulation on Cortical Spreading Depression Susceptibility and the Tissue Response in a Rat Model," *The Journal of Headache and Pain* 23, no. 1 (2022): 1–13.

78   Donald B. Hoover, "Cholinergic Modulation of the Immune System Presents New Approaches for Treating Inflammation," *Pharmacology & Therapeutics* 179 (2017): 1–16; Robert Kaczmarczyk, Dario Tejera, Bruce J. Simon, and Michael T. Heneka, "Microglia Modulation through External Vagus Nerve Stimulation in a Murine Model of Alzheimer's Disease," *Journal of Neurochemistry* 146, no. 1 (2018): 76–85; Javier Egea, et al., "Anti-Inflammatory Role of Microglial Alpha7 nAChRs and Its Role in Neuroprotection," *Biochemical Pharmacology* 97, no. 4 (2015): 463–472.

79   Esther Parada, et al., "The Microglial A7-Acetylcholine Nicotinic Receptor Is a Key Element in Promoting Neuroprotection by Inducing Heme Oxygenase-1 via Nuclear Factor Erythroid-2-Related Factor 2," *Antioxidants & Redox Signaling* 19, no. 11 (2013): 1135–1148; Ariana Q. Farrand, et al., "Vagus Nerve Stimulation Improves Locomotion and Neuronal Populations in a Model of Parkinson's Disease," *Brain Stimulation* 10, no. 6 (2017): 1045–1054; Stella Manta, Jianming Dong, Guy Debonnel, and Pierre Blier, "Enhancement of the Function of Rat Serotonin and Norepinephrine Neurons by Sustained Vagus Nerve Stimulation," *Journal of Psychiatry and Neuroscience* 34, no. 4 (2009): 272–280; JP Errico, "The Role of Vagus Nerve Stimulation in the Treatment of Central and Peripheral Pain Disorders and Related Comorbid Somatoform Conditions," *Neuromodulation* (2018): 1551–1564; Shih-Pin Chen, et al., "Vagus Nerve Stimulation Inhibits Cortical Spreading Depression," *Pain* 157, no. 4 (2016): 797; Hsiangkuo Yuan and Stephen D. Silberstein, "Vagus Nerve and Vagus Nerve Stimulation, a Comprehensive Review: Part III," *Headache: the Journal of Head and Face Pain* 56, no. 3 (2016): 479–490.

80   Graeme J. Gowans and D. Grahame Hardie, "AMPK: A Cellular Energy Sensor Primarily Regulated by AMP," (2014): 71–75; Shuai Jiang, et al., "AMPK: Potential Therapeutic Target for Ischemic Stroke," *Theranostics* 8, no. 16 (2018): 4535; Bharti Manwani and Louise D. McCullough,

"Function of the Master Energy Regulator Adenosine Monophosphate-Activated Protein Kinase in Stroke," *Journal of Neuroscience Research* 91, no. 8 (2013): 1018–1029.

81   Andre G. Douen, et al., "Preconditioning with Cortical Spreading Depression Decreases Intraischemic Cerebral Glutamate Levels and Down-Regulates Excitatory Amino Acid Transporters EAAT1 and EAAT2 from Rat Cerebral Cortex Plasma Membranes," *Journal of Neurochemistry* 75, no. 2 (2000): 812–818.

82   Ilknur Ay, Jie Lu, Hakan Ay, and A. Gregory Sorensen, "Vagus Nerve Stimulation Reduces Infarct Size in Rat Focal Cerebral Ischemia," *Neuroscience Letters* 459, no. 3 (2009): 147–151.

83   Ilknur Ay, Rena Nasser, Bruce Simon, and Hakan Ay, "Transcutaneous Cervical Vagus Nerve Stimulation Ameliorates Acute Ischemic Injury in Rats," *Brain Stimulation* 9, no. 2 (2016): 166–173.

84   Yirong Yang, et al., "Non-Invasive Vagus Nerve Stimulation Reduces Blood-Brain Barrier Disruption in a Rat Model of Ischemic Stroke," *Brain Stimulation* 11, no. 4 (2018): 689–698.

85   Bin Zhou, Pablo Perel, George A. Mensah, and Majid Ezzati, "Global Epidemiology, Health Burden, and Effective Interventions for Elevated Blood Pressure and Hypertension," *Nature Reviews Cardiology* 18, no. 11 (2021): 785–802.

86   Bin Zhou, Pablo Perel, George A. Mensah, and Majid Ezzati, "Global Epidemiology, Health Burden and Effective Interventions for Elevated Blood Pressure and Hypertension," *Nature Reviews Cardiology* 18, no. 11 (2021): 785–802.

87   Tomoaki Suzuki, et al., "Noninvasive Vagus Nerve Stimulation Prevents Ruptures and Improves Outcomes in a Model of Intracranial Aneurysm in Mice," *Stroke* 50, no. 5 (2019): 1216–1223.

88   Suzuki, et al., "Noninvasive Vagus Nerve Stimulation Prevents Ruptures."

89   Mayo Clinic, "Metabolic Syndrome," *Mayo Clinic,* May 6, 2021, https://www.mayoclinic.org/diseases-conditions/metabolic-syndrome/symptoms-causes/syc-20351916.

90   National Heart, Lung, and Blood Institute, "What Is Metabolic Syndrome?" Accessed October 19, 2023, https://www.nhlbi.nih.gov/health/metabolic-syndrome.

91   John Hopkins Medicine, "Metabolic Syndrome," Hopkins Medicine, Accessed October 19, 2023, https://www.hopkinsmedicine.org/health /conditions-and-diseases/metabolic-syndrome; Engin, "The Definition and Prevalence of Obesity and Metabolic Syndrome," *Advances in Experimental Medicine and Biology* 960 (2017): 1–17.

92   Afshin, et al., "Health Effects of Overweight and Obesity in 195 Countries over 25 Years," *The New England Journal of Medicine* 377 (2017): 13–27.

93   Lakka, et al., "The Metabolic Syndrome and Total and Cardiovascular Disease Mortality in Middle-aged Men," *JAMA* 288, no. 21 (2002): 2709–2716.

94   Yuri Milaneschi, W. Kyle Simmons, Elisabeth FC van Rossum, and Brenda W. J. H. Penninx, "Depression and Obesity: Evidence of Shared Biological Mechanisms," *Molecular Psychiatry* 24, no. 1 (2019): 18–33; Weonjeong Lim, Suzi Hong, Richard Nelesen, and Joel E. Dimsdale, "The Association of Obesity, Cytokine Levels, And Depressive Symptoms with Diverse Measures of Fatigue in Healthy Subjects," *Archives of Internal Medicine* 165, no. 8 (2005): 910–915.

95   Abhishek K. Jha, et al., "Network Integration of Parallel Metabolic and Transcriptional Data Reveals Metabolic Modules That Regulate Macrophage Polarization," *Immunity* 42, (2015): 419–430.

96   Florido, et al., "Melatonin Drives Apoptosis in Head and Neck Cancer by Increasing Mitochondrial ROS Generated via Reverse Electron Transport," *Journal of Pineal Research* 73, no. 3 (2022): E12824; Sten Orrenius and Boris Zhivotovsky, "Cardiolipin Oxidation Sets Cytochrome *C* Free," *Nature Chemical Biology* 1 (2005): 188–189 https://doi.org/10.1038 /Nchembio0905-188; Melhuish Lindsay M. Melhuish Beaupre, et al., "Melatonin's Neuroprotective Role in Mitochondria and Its Potential as a Biomarker in Aging, Cognition, and Psychiatric Disorders," *Translational Psychiatry* 11 (2021): 339.

97   Christopher K. Glass and Gioacchino Natoli, "Molecular Control of Activation and Priming in Macrophages," *Nature Immunology* 17, no. 1 (2015): 26–33.

98   Kohjiro Ueki, et al., "Suppressor of Cytokine Signaling 1 (SOCS-1) and SOCS-3 Cause Insulin Resistance through Inhibition of Tyrosine Phosphorylation of Insulin Receptor Substrate Proteins by Discrete Mechanisms," *Molecular and Cellular Biology* 24, no. 12: 5434–5446.

99 XianFeng Wang, et al., "Activation of the Cholinergic Antiinflammatory Pathway Ameliorates Obesity-Induced inflammation and Insulin Resistance," *Endocrinology* 152 (2011): 836–846.

100 S. Shikora, et al., "Vagal Blocking Improves Glycemic Control and Elevated Blood Pressure in Obese Subjects with Type 2 Diabetes Mellitus," *Journal of Obesity* (2013).

101 Lebovitz, et al., "Treatment of Patients with Obese Type 2 Diabetes with Tantalus-DIAMOND® Gastric Electrical Stimulation: Normal Triglycerides Predict Durable Effects for at Least 3 Years," *Hormone and Metabolic Research* 47 (2015): 456–462.

102 Shai Policker, et al., "Treatment of Type 2 Diabetes Using Meal-Triggered Gastric Electrical Stimulation," *Israel Medical Association World Fellowship Conference* 11 (2009): 206–208; Lebovitz, et al., "Treatment of Patients with Obese Type 2 Diabetes; Hans-Rudolf Berthoud, et al., "Vagal Mechanisms as Neuromodulatory Targets for the Treatment of Metabolic Disease," *Annals of the New York Academy of Sciences* 1454 (2019): 42–55.

103 Jin-Zhou Zhu, et al., "Prevalence of Nonalcoholic Fatty Liver Disease and Economy," *Digestive Diseases and Sciences* 60 (2015): 3194–3202.

104 Kumi Kimura, et al., "Central Insulin Action Activates Kupffer Cells by Suppressing Hepatic Vagal Activation via the Nicotinic Alpha 7 Acetylcholine Receptor," *Cell Reports* 14 (2016): 2362–2374.

105 Takahiro Nishio, et al., "Hepatic Vagus Nerve Regulates Kupffer Cell Activation via A7 Nicotinic Acetylcholine Receptor in Nonalcoholic Steatohepatitis," *Journal of Gastroenterology* 52, no.8 (2017): 965–976.

106 Dong-Jie Li, et al., "Nicotinic Acetylcholine Receptor A7 Subunit Improves Energy Homeostasis and Inhibits Inflammation in Nonalcoholic Fatty Liver Disease," *Metabolism* 79 (2018): 52–63.

107 Victoria Fernandez-Garcia, et al., "Contribution of Extramedullary Hematopoiesis to Atherosclerosis. The Spleen as a Neglected Hub of Inflammatory Cells," *Frontiers in Immunology* 11, (2020): 586527.

108 Daniela Flores-Gomez, et al., "Trained Immunity in Atherosclerotic Cardiovascular Disease," *Current Opinion in Lipidology* 30, no. 5 (2019): 395–400.

109   Jody Tori O. Cabrera and Ayako Makino, "Efferocytosis of Vascular Cells in Cardiovascular Disease," *Pharmacological therapeutics* 229 (2022): 107919.

110   Yoko Kojima, et al., "The Role of Efferocytosis in Atherosclerosis," *Circulation* 135, no. 5 (2017): 476–489.

111   Cabrera and Makino, "Efferocytosis of Vascular Cells in Cardiovascular Disease," *Pharmacological Therapeutics* 229 (2022): 107919.

112   Peter Libby, "History of Discovery: Inflammation in Atherosclerosis, Arteriosclerosis Thrombosis and Vascular Biology," *Arterioscler Thromb Vasc Biology* 32, no. 9 (2012): 2045–2051.

113   Anastasia Poznyak, et al., "The Diabetes Mellitus–Atherosclerosis Connection: The Role of Lipid and Glucose Metabolism and Chronic Inflammation," *International Journal of Molecular Sciences* 21 (2020): 1835.

114   Zhengjiang Qian, et al., "The Cholinergic Anti-Inflammatory Pathway Attenuates the Development of Atherosclerosis in Apoe-/- Mice through Modulating Macrophage Functions," *Biomedicines* 9 (2021): 1150; Ildernandes Vieira-Alves, et al., "Role of the a7 Nicotinic Acetylcholine Receptor in the Pathophysiology of Atherosclerosis," *Frontiers in Physiology* 11 (2020): 621769.

115   Daniela Matei, et al., "Impact of Non-Pharmacological Interventions on the Mechanisms of Atherosclerosis," *International Journal of Molecular Sciences* 23, no. 16 (2022): 9097.

116   Sailesh C. Harwani, "Macrophages Under Pressure: The Role of Macrophage Polarization in Hypertension," *Translational Research* 191 (2018): 45–63.

117   Shu-Zhong Jiang, et al., "Obesity and Hypertension," *Experimental and Therapeutic Medicine* 12, no. 4 (2016): 2395–2399.

118   Alfonso Eirin, et al., "Mitochondria: A Pathogenic Paradigm in Hypertensive Renal Disease," *Hypertension* 65, no. 2 (2015): 264–270; Jeffrey D. Marshall, et al., "Mitochondrial Dysfunction and Pulmonary Hypertension: Cause, Effect, or Both," *American Journal of Physiology-Lung Cellular and Molecular Physiology* 314 no. 5 (2018): L782-L796.

119   Elizabeth M. Annoni, et al., "Intermittent Electrical Stimulation of the Right Cervical Vagus Nerve in Salt-Sensitive Hypertensive

Rats: Effects on Blood Pressure, Arrhythmias, and Ventricular Electrophysiology," *Physiological Reports* 3, no. 8 (2015): e12476.

120   Policker, et al., "Treatment of Type 2 Diabetes."

121   Shikora, et al., "Vagal Blocking Improves Glycemic Control."

122   Yi-Gang Chen, "Research Progress in the Pathogenesis of Alzheimer's Disease," *Chinese Medical Journal* 131 (2018): 1618–24.

123   Robert W. Mahley, Karl H. Weisgraber, and Yadong Huang, "Apolipoprotein E4: A Causative Factor and therapeutic Target in Neuropathology, Including Alzheimer's Disease," *Proceedings of the National Academy of Sciences* 103, no. 15 (2006): 5644–5651.

124   Anushka Chakravorty, et al., "Dysfunctional Mitochondria and Mitophagy as Drivers of Alzheimer's Disease Pathogenesis," *Frontiers in Aging Neuroscience* 11 (2019): 311; Bhargavi Kulkarni, Natália Cruz-Martins, and Dileep Kumar, "Microglia in Alzheimer's Disease: An Unprecedented Opportunity as Prospective Drug Target," *Molecular Neurobiology* 59, no. 5 (2022): 2678–2693 (2022).

125   Eric Steen, et al., "Impaired Insulin and Insulin-Like Growth Factor Expression and Signaling Mechanisms in Alzheimer's Disease—Is This Type 3 Diabetes?" *Journal of Alzheimer's Disease* 7, no. 1 (2005): 63–80 (2005)

126   E. Rönnemaa, et al., "Impaired Insulin Secretion Increases the Risk of Alzheimer Disease," *Neurology* 71 (2008) 1065–1071.

127   Ramesh Kandimalla, Vani Thirumala, P. Hemachandra Reddy, "Is Alzheimer's Disease a Type 3 Diabetes? A Critical Appraisal," *Biochimica Et Biophysica Actait* 1863, (2017): 1078–1089; Suzanne de la Monte and Ming Tong, "Brain Metabolic Dysfunction at the Core of Alzheimer's Disease," *Biochemical Pharmacology* 88, no. 4 (2014): 548–559.

128   Robert Kaczmarczyk, Dario Tejera, Bruce J. Simon, and Michael T. Heneka, "Microglia Modulation through External Vagus " *Journal of Neurochemistry* 146, no. 1 (2018): 76–85; Ilknur Ay, Rena Nasser, Bruce Simon, and Hakan Ay, "Transcutaneous Cervical Vagus Nerve Stimulation Ameliorates Acute Ischemic Injury in Rats," *Brain Stimulation* 9, no. 2, (2016): 166–173; Jordan L. Hawkins, Lauren E. Cornelison, Brian A. Blankenship, and Paul L. Durham, "Vagus Nerve Stimulation Inhibits Trigeminal Nociception in a Rodent Model of Episodic Migraine," *Pain Reports* 2 (2017): 6; Magnus J. C. Sjorgen, et al., "Cognition-Enhancing Effect of Vagus Nerve Stimulation in Patients with Alzheimer's Disease:

A Pilot Study," *Journal of Clinical Psychiatry* 63, no. 11 (2002): 972–980; Charley A. Merrill, et al., "Vagus Nerve Stimulation in Patients with Alzheimer's Disease: Additional Follow-Up Results of a Pilot Study through 1 Year," *Journal of Clinical Psychiatry* 67, no. 8 (2006): 1171–1178.

129   L. L. Espey, "Ovulation as an Inflammatory Reaction—A Hypothesis," *Biology of Reproduction* 22, no. 1 (1980): 73–106 (1980); Diane M. Duffy, et al., "Ovulation: Parallels with Inflammatory Processes," *Endocrine Reviews* 40 (2019): 369– 416.

130   C. D. Kuo, et al., "Biphasic Changes in Autonomic Nervous Activity during Pregnancy," *British Journal of Anaesthesia* 84, no. 3 (2000): 323–329.

131   Khalida Itriyeva, "Premenstrual Syndrome and Premenstrual Dysphoric Disorder in Adolescents," *Current Problems in Pediatric and Adolescent Health Care* 52 (2022): 101187.

132   Lara Tiranini and Rossella E. Nappi, "Recent Advances in Understanding/Management of Premenstrual Dysphoric Disorder/ Premenstrual Syndrome," *Faculty Reviews* 11, no. 11 (2022); Sabrina Hofmeister, and Seth Bodden, "Premenstrual Syndrome and Premenstrual Dysphoric Disorder," *American Family Physician* 94, no. 3 (2016): 236–240.

133   Nicole Lichtblau, et al., "Cytokines as Biomarkers in Depressive Disorder: Current Standing and Prospects," *International Review of Psychiatry* 25, no. 5 (2013): 592–603; Sandra Malynn, Antonio Campos-Torres, Paul Moynagh, and Jana Haase "The Pro-Inflammatory Cytokine TNF-A Regulates the Activity and Expression of the Serotonin Transporter (SERT) in Astrocytes," *Neurochemical Research* 38 (2013): 694–704.

134   Zijing Zhang, Lu Huang, Lynae Brayboy, "Macrophages: An Indispensable Piece of Ovarian Health," *Biology of Reproduction* (2020): 1–12.

135   Ellen B. Gold, Craig Wells, and Marianne O'Neill Rasor, "The Association of Inflammation with Premenstrual Symptoms," *Journal of Women's Health* 25, no. 9 (2016): 865–874.

136   Şadan Yazar and Mehmet Yazıcı, "Impact of Menstrual Cycle on Cardiac Autonomic Function Assessed by Heart Rate Variability and Heart Rate Recovery," *Medical Principles and Practice* 25, no. 4 (2016):

374–377; Rama Choudhury, et al., "Sympathetic Nerve Function Status in Follicular and Late Luteal Phases of Menstrual Cycle in Healthy Young Women," *Journal of Bangladesh Society of Physiologist* 5, no. 2 (2010): 80–88.

137   Georg Pongratz and Rainer H. Straub, "The Sympathetic Nervous Response in Inflammation," *Arthritis Research & Therapy* 16 (2014): 1–12; Tamaki Matsumoto, et al., "Altered Autonomic Nervous System Activity as a Potential Etiological Factor of Premenstrual Syndrome and Premenstrual Dysphoric Disorder," *Biopsychosocial Medicine* 1 (2007): 24.

138   Hikmet Yorgun, et al., "Evaluation of Cardiac Autonomic Function by Various Indices in Patients with Primary Premature Ovarian Failure," *Clinical Research in Cardiology* 101 (2012): 753–759.

139   Leah M. Jappe, et al., "Stress and Eating Disorder Behavior in Anorexia Nervosa as a Function of Menstrual Cycle Status," *International Journal of Eating Disorders* 47, no. 2 (2014): 181–188; Suvi Ravi, et al., "Self-Reported Restrictive Eating, Eating Disorders, Menstrual Dysfunction, and Injuries in Athletes Competing at Different Levels and Sports," *Nutrients* 13, no. 9 (2021): 3275.

140   Dong-mei Huang, et al., "Acupuncture for Infertility: Is It an Effective Therapy?" *Chinese Journal of Integrative Medicine* 17, no. 5 (2011): 386–395.

141   Ayu Cintani Kusuma, et al., "Electroacupuncture Enhances Number of Mature Oocytes and Fertility Rates for In Vitro Fertilization," *Medical Acupuncture* 31, no. 5 (2019): 289–297.

142   Shike Zhang, et al., "Transcutaneous Auricular Vagus Nerve Stimulation as a Potential Novel Treatment for Polycystic Ovary Syndrome," *Scientific Reports* 13, no. 1 (2023): 7721.

143   Polly Fu, et al., "Anxiety, Depressive Symptoms, and Cardiac Autonomic Function in Perimenopausal and Postmenopausal Women with Hot Flashes: A Brief Report," *Menopause* 25, no. 12 (2018): 1470–1475.

144   Robert R. Freedman, Michael L. Kruger, and Samuel L. Wasson, "Heart Rate Variability in Menopausal Hot Flashes during Sleep," *Menopause* 18, no. 8 (2011): 897–900; Jin Oh Lee, et al., "The Relationship Between Menopausal Symptoms and Heart Rate Variability in Middle Aged Women," *Korean Journal of Family Medicine* 32 (2011): 299–305; Massimiliano de Zambotti, "Vagal Withdrawal during Hot Flashes

Occurring in Undisturbed Sleep: Hot Flashes and Autonomic Activity," *Menopause* 20, no. 11 (2013).

145   Wan-Yu Huang, et al., "Circulating Interleukin-8 and Tumor Necrosis Factor-A Are Associated with Hot Flashes in Healthy Postmenopausal Women," *PloS One* 12, no. 8 (2017): E0184011; Robert R. Freedman, Michael L. Kruger, and Samuel L. Wasson, "Heart Rate Variability in Menopausal Hot Flashes during Sleep," *Menopause* 18, no. 8 (2011): 897.

146   T. Ivarsson, A. C. Spetz, and M. Hammar, "Physical Exercise and Vasomotor Symptoms in Postmenopausal Women," *Maturitas* 29, no. 2 (1998): 139–46; Tom G. Bailey, et al., "Exercise Training Reduces the Frequency of Menopausal Hot by Improving Thermoregulatory Control," *Menopause* 23, no. 7 (2016): 708–718; Janet S. Carpenter, "Physical Activity Is Not a Recommended Treatment for Hot Flashes," *Menopause* 30, no. 2 (2023): 121; Sarah Witkowski, et al., "Physical Activity and Exercise for Hot Flashes: Trigger or Treatment?" *Menopause* 30, no. 2 (2023): 10-1097.

147   Min-Kyu Sung, et al., "A Potential Association of Meditation with Menopausal Symptoms and Blood Chemistry in Healthy Women: A Pilot Cross-Sectional Study," *Medicine* 99, no. 36 (2020).

148   Naglaa Fathy Fathalla Zaied, et al., "Effect of Paced Breathing Technique on Hot Flashes and Quality of Daily Life Activities among Surgically Menopaused Women," *Egyptian Journal of Health Care* 10, no. 4 (2019).

149   Christina Brock, et al., "Transcutaneous Cervical Vagal Nerve Stimulation Modulates Cardiac Vagal Tone and Tumor Necrosis Factor-Alpha," *Neurogastroenterology and Motility* 29, no. 5 (2017): E12999; Tyvin Rich, et al., "Intermittent 96-Hour Auricular Electroacupuncture for Hot Flashes in Patients with Prostate Cancer: A Pilot Study," *Medical Acupuncture* 29, no. 5, (2017): 313–321.

150   Scott M. Berry, et al., "A Patient-Level Meta-Analysis of Studies Evaluating Vagus Nerve Stimulation Therapy for Treatment-Resistant Depression," *Medical Devices: Evidence and Research* (2013): 17–35; Mark S. George, et al., "A Pilot Study of Vagus Nerve Stimulation (VNS) for Treatment-Resistant Anxiety Disorders," *Brain Stimulation* 1, no. 2 (2008): 112–121.

151   Katherine A. Stamatakis and Naresh M. Punjabi, "Effects of Sleep Fragmentation on Glucose Metabolism in Normal Subjects," *Chest* 137, no. 1 (2010): 95–101.

152   Michael R. Irwin, "Sleep Disruption Induces Activation of Inflammation and Heightens Risk for Infectious Disease: Role of Impairments in Thermoregulation and Elevated Ambient Temperature," *Temperature* 10, no. 2 (2023): 198–234.

153   Tove Hallböök, et al., "Beneficial Effects on Sleep of Vagus Nerve Stimulation in Children with Therapy Resistant Epilepsy," *European Journal of Paediatric Neurology* 9, no. 6 (2005): 399–407

154   Elena Zambrelli, et al., "Laryngeal Motility Alteration: A Missing Link between Sleep Apnea and Vagus Nerve Stimulation for Epilepsy," *Epilepsia* 57, no. 1 (2016): E24–E27

155   Jessica Tarn, et al., "The Effects of Noninvasive Vagus Nerve Stimulation on Fatigue in Participants with Primary Sjögren's Syndrome," *Neuromodulation: Technology at the Neural Interface* 26, no. 3 (2023): 681–689.

156   Emily D. Szmuilowicz, et al., "Vasomotor Symptoms and Cardiovascular Events in Postmenopausal Women," *Menopause* 18, no. 6 (2011): 63; Dongshan Zhu, et al., "Vasomotor Menopausal Symptoms and Risk of Cardiovascular Disease: A Pooled Analysis of Six Prospective Studies," *American Journal of Obstetrics & Gynecology* 223 no. 6 (2020): 898; Aris Bechlioulis et al., "Increased Vascular Inflammation in Early Menopausal Women Is Associated with Hot Flush Severity," *The Journal of Clinical Endocrinology & Metabolism* 97, no. 5 (2012): E760 –E764; Wan-Yu Huang, et al., "Circulating Interleukin-8 and Tumor Necrosis Factor-α Are Associated with Hot Flashes in Healthy Postmenopausal Women," *PloS One* 12, no. 8 (2017); N. Biglia, et al., "Vasomotor Symptoms in Menopause: A Biomarker of Cardiovascular Disease Risk," *Climacteric* 20, no. 4 (2017): 306–312; Roisin Worsley, et al., "Moderate-Severe Vasomotor Symptoms Are Associated with Moderate-Severe Depressive Symptoms," *Journal of Women's Health* 26, no. 7 (2017); Lauren L. Drogos, et al., "Objective Cognitive Performance Is Related to Subjective Memory Complaints in Midlife Women with Moderate to Severe Vasomotor Symptoms," *Menopause* 20, no. 12 (2013).

157   N. Biglia, et al., "Vasomotor Symptoms in Menopause: A Biomarker of Cardiovascular Disease Risk," *Climacteric*, 20, no. 4 (August 2017): 306-312, doi: 10.1080/13697137.2017.1315089.

158   Feng Ma, et al., "Effects of a7nAChR Agonist on the Tissue Estrogen Receptor Expression of Castrated Rats," *International Journal of Clinical and Experimental* Pathology 8 no. 10 (2015): 13421–13425.

159   Roisin Worsley, et al., "Moderate-Severe Vasomotor Symptoms Are Associated with Moderate-Severe Depressive Symptoms," *Journal of Women's Health* 26, no. 7 (2017): 712–718; Martha Hickey, C. Bryant, and F. Judd, "Evaluation and Management of Depressive and Anxiety Symptoms in Midlife," *Climacteric* 15, no. 1 (2012): 3–9; Angelo Cagnacci, et al., "Menopausal Symptoms and Risk Factors for Cardiovascular Disease in Postmenopause," *Climacteric* 15, no. 2 (2012): 157–162.

160   G. M. C. Rosano, C. Vitale, G. Marazzi, and M. Volterrani, "Menopause and Cardiovascular Disease: The Evidence," *Climacteric* 10, no. 1 (2007): 19–24; J. J. Von Holzen, G. Capaldo, Matthias Wilhelm, and Petra Stute, "Impact of Endo- and Exogenous Estrogens on Heart Rate Variability in Women: A Review," *Climacteric* 19, no. 3 (2016): 222–228; Ki-Jin Ryu, et al., "Vasomotor Symptoms: More Than Temporary Menopausal Symptoms," *Journal of Menopausal Medicine* 26, no. 3 (2020): 147.

161   Taulant Muka, et al., "Association of Vasomotor and Other Menopausal Symptoms with Risk of Cardiovascular Disease: A Systematic Review and Meta-Analysis," *PloS One* 11, no. 6 (2016): e0157417; Polly Fu, et al., "Anxiety, Depressive Symptoms, and Cardiac Autonomic Function in Perimenopausal and Postmenopausal Women with Hot Flashes: A Brief Report," *Menopause* 25, no. 12 (2018): 1470–1475.

162   Jacqueline Pesa and Maureen J. Lage, "The Medical Costs of Migraine and Comorbid Anxiety and Depression," *Headache: The Journal of Head and Face Pain* 44, no. 6 (2004): 562–570; Muhammad B. Yunus, "Role of Central Sensitization in Symptoms Beyond Muscle Pain, and the Evaluation of a Patient with Widespread Pain," *Best Practice & Research Clinical Rheumatology* 21, no. 3 (2007): 481–497.

163   Anil K. Seth, "Interoceptive Inference, Emotion, and the Embodied self," *Trends in Cognitive Sciences* 17, no. 11 (2013): 565–573.

164   Jo Nijs, et al., "Brain-Derived Neurotrophic Factor as a Driving Force behind Neuroplasticity in Neuropathic and Central Sensitization

Pain: A New Therapeutic Target?" *Expert Opinion on Therapeutic Targets* 19, no. 4 (2015): 565–576.

165   Clifford J. Woolf, "Recent Advances in the Pathophysiology of Acute Pain," *British Journal of Anaesthesia* 63, no. 2 (1989): 139–146; Clifford J. Woolf, "What Is This Thing Called Pain?" *The Journal of Clinical Investigation* 120, no. 11 (2010): 3742–3744.

166   Sarah C. P. Williams, "Epigenetics," *Proceedings of the National Academy of Sciences* 110, no. 9 (2013): 3209–3209.

167   Mikhail Spivakov and Amanda G. Fisher, "Epigenetic Signatures of Stem-Cell Identity," *Nature Reviews Genetics* 8, no. 4 (2007): 263–271; C. David Allis and Thomas Jenuwein, "The Molecular Hallmarks of Epigenetic Control," *Nature Reviews Genetics* 17, no. 8 (2016): 487–500.

168   Alexandra L. Mattei, Nina Bailly, and Alexander Meissner, "DNA Methylation: A Historical Perspective," *Trends in Genetics* 38, no. 7 (2022): 676–707.

169   Grigoriy A. Armeev, et al., "Histone Dynamics Mediate DNA Unwrapping and Sliding in Nucleosomes," *Nature Communications* 12, no. 1 (2021): 2387; Sari Pennings, Geert Meersseman, and E. Morton Bradbury, "Linker Histones H1 and H5 Prevent the Mobility of Positioned Nucleosomes," *Proceedings of the National Academy of Sciences* 91, no. 22 (1994): 10275–10279.

170   Carmen Brenner and François Fuks, "A Methylation Rendezvous: Reader Meets Writers," *Developmental Cell* 12, no. 6 (2007): 843–844; Heng Zhu, Guohua Wang, and Jiang Qian, "Transcription Factors as Readers and Effectors of DNA Methylation," *Nature Reviews Genetics* 17, no. 9 (2016): 551–565.

171   Adrian P. Bird, "Methyl-CpG Islands as Gene Markers in the Vertebrate Nucleus," *Trends in Genetics* 3 (1987): 342–347; Joseph L. McClay, et al., "A Methylome-Wide Study of Aging Using Massively Parallel Sequencing of the Methyl-CpG-Enriched Genomic Fraction from Blood in Over 700 Subjects," *Human Molecular Genetics* 23, no. 5 (2014): 1175–1185; Daniel F. Schorderet and Stanley M. Gartler, "Analysis of CpG Suppression in Methylated and Nonmethylated Species," *Proceedings of the National Academy of Sciences* 89, no. 3 (1992): 957–961.

172   Aimée M. Deaton and Adrian Bird, "CpG Islands and the Regulation of Transcription," *Genes & Development* 25, no. 10 (2011): 1010–1022; Robert S. Illingworth and Adrian P. Bird, "CpG Islands—'A Rough Guide,'"

FEBS Letters 583, no. 11 (2009): 1713–1720; Francisco Antequera, "Structure, Function, and Evolution of CpG Island Promoters," *Cellular and Molecular Life Sciences* 60 (2003): 1647–1658; Sari Pennings, James Allan, and Colin S. Davey, "DNA Methylation, Nucleosome Formation, and Positioning," *Briefings in Functional Genomics* 3, no. 4 (2005): 351–361.

173   Pier-Luc Clermont, Abhijit Parolia, Hui Hsuan Liu, and Cheryl D. Helgason, "DNA Methylation at Enhancer Regions: Novel Avenues for Epigenetic Biomarker Development," *Frontiers in Bioscience-Landmark* 21, no. 2 (2016): 430–446; Robert S. Illingworth, et al., "Orphan CpG Islands Identify Numerous Conserved Promoters in the Mammalian Genome," *Plos Genetics* 6, no. 9 (2010): E1001134.

174   Hideyuki Takeshima, et al., "TET Repression and Increased DNMT Activity Synergistically Induce Aberrant DNA Methylation," *The Journal of Clinical Investigation* 130, no. 10 (2020): 5370–5379; Else Eising, Nicole A. Datson, Arn M. J. M. Van Den Maagdenberg, and Michel D. Ferrari, "Epigenetic Mechanisms in Migraine: A Promising Avenue?" *BMC Medicine* 11 (2013): 1–6; Laura S. Stone and Moshe Szyf, "The Emerging Field of Pain Epigenetics," *Pain* 154, no. 1 (2013): 1–2; Marta Kulis and Manel Esteller, "DNA Methylation and Cancer," *Advances in Genetics* 70 (2010): 27–56.

175   Bruce S. Hass, et al., "Effects of Caloric Restriction in Animals on Cellular Function, Oncogene Expression, and DNA Methylation In Vitro," *Mutation Research/Dnaging* 295, no. 4–6 (1993): 281–289; Meeshanthini Vijayendran, et al., "Effects of Genotype and Child Abuse on DNA Methylation and Gene Expression at the Serotonin Transporter," *Frontiers in Psychiatry* 3 (2012): 55; Mirian Samblas, Fermín I. Milagro, and Alfredo Martínez, "DNA Methylation Markers in Obesity, Metabolic Syndrome, and Weight Loss," *Epigenetics* 14, no. 5 (2019): 421–444; Adam E. Field, et al., "DNA Methylation Clocks in Aging: Categories, Causes, And Consequences," *Molecular Cell* 71, no. 6 (2018): 882–895; Axel Kowald, "The Mitochondrial Theory of Aging," *Neurosignals* 10, no. 3–4 (2001): 162–175.

176   Wei Jiang, et al., "DNA Methylation: A Target in Neuropathic Pain," *Frontiers in Medicine* 9 (2022): 879902; Lingli Liang, Brianna Marie Lutz, Alex Bekker, and Yuan-Xiang Tao, "Epigenetic Regulation of Chronic Pain," *Epigenomics* 7, no. 2 (2015): 235–245; Judit Garriga, et al., "Nerve Injury-Induced Chronic Pain Is Associated with Persistent DNA Methylation Reprogramming in Dorsal Root Ganglion," *Journal of Neuroscience* 38, no. 27 (2018): 6090–610.

177   Elmar W. Tobi, et al., "DNA Methylation Signatures Link Prenatal Famine Exposure to Growth and Metabolism," *Nature Communications* 5, no. 1 (2014): 5592.

178   Rachel Yehuda, et al., "Holocaust Exposure Induced Intergenerational Effects on FKBP5 Methylation," *Biological Psychiatry* 80, no. 5 (2016): 372–380.

179   Roy S. Wu, Henryk T. Panusz, Christopher L. Hatch, and William M. Bonner, "Histones and Their Modification," *Critical Reviews in Biochemistry* 20, no. 2 (1986): 201–263; Artemi Bendandi, Alessandro S. Patelli, Alberto Diaspro, and Walter Rocchia, "The Role of Histone Tails in Nucleosome Stability: An Electrostatic Perspective," *Computational and Structural Biotechnology Journal* 18 (2020): 2799–2809.

180   Hiroshi Kimura, "Histone Modifications for Human Epigenome Analysis," *Journal of Human Genetics* 58, no. 7 (2013): 439–445.

181   Alison L. Clayton, Catherine A. Hazzalin, and Louis C. Mahadevan, "Enhanced Histone Acetylation and Transcription: A Dynamic Perspective," *Molecular Cell* 23, no. 3 (2006): 289–296; Palak Gujral, Vishakha Mahajan, Abbey C. Lissaman, and Anna P. Ponnampalam, "Histone Acetylation and the Role of Histone Deacetylases in Normal Cyclic Endometrium," *Reproductive Bio and Endocrinology* 18 (2020): 1–11; Santiago Ropero and Manel Esteller, "The Role of Histone Deacetylases (Hdacs) in Human Cancer," *Molecular Oncology* 1, no. 1 (2007): 19–25.

182   Ashwini Jambhekar, Abhinav Dhall, and Yang Shi, "Roles and Regulation of Histone Methylation in Animal Development," *Nature Reviews Molecular Cell Biology* 20, no. 10 (2019): 625–641; Robert J. Sims, and Danny Reinberg, "Histone H3 Lys 4 Methylation: Caught in a Bind?" *Genes & Development* 20, no. 20 (2006): 2779–2786.

183   Emily L. Putiri and Keith D. Robertson, "Epigenetic Mechanisms and Genome Stability," *Clinical Epigenetics* 2 (2011): 299–314; Thomas Schalch, et al., "High-Affinity Binding of Chp1 Chromodomain to K9 Methylated Histone H3 Is Required to Establish Centromeric Heterochromatin," *Molecular Cell* 34, no. 1 (2009): 36–46; Benjamin D. Towbin, et al., "Step-Wise Methylation of Histone H3K9 Positions Heterochromatin at the Nuclear Periphery," *Cell* 150, no. 5 (2012): 934–947.

184   Ali Shilatifard, "Molecular Implementation and Physiological Roles for Histone H3 Lysine 4 (H3K4) Methylation," *Current Opinion in Cell Biology* 20, no. 3 (2008): 341–348.

185 Ali Shilatifard, "The COMPASS Family of Histone H3K4 Methylases: Mechanisms of Regulation in Development and Disease Pathogenesis," *Annual Review of Biochemistry* 81 (2012): 65–95.

186 Ali Sharifi-Zarchi, et al., "DNA Methylation Regulates Discrimination of Enhancers from Promoters through a H3K4me1-H3K4me3 Seesaw Mechanism," *BMC Genomics* 18 (2017): 1–21.

187 Terrence J. Monks, Ruiyu Xie, Kulbhushan Tikoo, and Serrine S. Lau, "Ros-Induced Histone Modifications and Their Role in Cell Survival and Cell Death," *Drug Metabolism Reviews* 38, no. 4 (2006): 755–767; Maria Ninova, Katalin Fejes Tóth, and Alexei A. Aravin, "The Control of Gene Expression and Cell Identity by H3K9 Trimethylation," *Development* 146, no. 19 (2019): Dev181180.

188 Kirsty Jamieson, et al., "Loss of HP1 Causes Depletion of H3k27me3 from Facultative Heterochromatin and Gain of H3K27me2 at Constitutive Heterochromatin," *Genome Research* 26, no. 1 (2016): 97–107; Lianying Jiao, and Xin Liu, "Structural Basis of Histone H3K27 Trimethylation by an Active Polycomb Repressive Complex 2," *Science* 350, no. 6258 (2015): Aac4383; James P. Reddington, et al., "Redistribution of H3K27me3 Upon DNA Hypomethylation Results in De-Repression of Polycomb Target Genes," *Genome Biology* 14 (2013): 1–17; Joanna Boros, et al.,"Polycomb Repressive Complex 2 and H3K27me3 Cooperate with H3K9 Methylation to Maintain Heterochromatin Protein 1α at Chromatin," *Molecular and Cellular Biology* 34, no. 19 (2014): 3662–3674; Kai Ge, "Epigenetic Regulation of Adipogenesis by Histone Methylation," *Biochimica Et Biophysica Acta (BBA)-Gene Regulatory Mechanisms* 1819, no. 7 (2012): 727–732; Paul Chammas, Ivano Mocavini, and Luciano Di Croce, "Engaging Chromatin: PRC2 Structure Meets Function," *British Journal of Cancer* 122, no. 3 (2020): 315–328; Neil Justin, et al., "Structural Basis of Oncogenic Histone H3K27M Inhibition of Human Polycomb Repressive Complex 2," *Nature Communications* 7, no. 1 (2016): 11316.

189 Karin J. Ferrari, et al., "Polycomb-Dependent H3K27me1 and H3K27me2 Regulate Active Transcription and Enhancer Fidelity," *Molecular Cell* 53, no. 1 (2014): 49–62; Aster H. Juan, et al., "Roles of H3K27me2 And H3KL27me3 Examined during Fate Specification of Embryonic Stem Cells," *Cell Reports* 17, no. 5 (2016): 1369–1382.

190   Yingying Lin, et al., "Role of Histone Post-Translational Modifications in Inflammatory Diseases," *Frontiers in Immunology* 13 (2022): 852272.

191   Irfan Rahman, Peter S. Gilmour, Luis Albert Jimenez, and William Macnee, "Oxidative Stress and TNF-A Induce Histone Acetylation and NF-Kb/AP-1 Activation in Alveolar Epithelial Cells: Potential Mechanism in Gene Transcription in Lung Inflammation," *Oxygen/Nitrogen Radicals: Cell Injury and Disease* (2002): 239-248; Maria G. Daskalaki, Christos Tsatsanis, and Sotirios C. Kampranis, "Histone Methylation and Acetylation in Macrophages as a Mechanism for Regulation of Inflammatory Responses," *Journal of Cellular Physiology* 233, no. 9 (2018): 6495-6507.

192   Amy Guillaumet-Adkins, et al., "Epigenetics and Oxidative Stress in Aging," *Oxidative Medicine and Cellular Longevity* (2017).

193   Yingmei Niu, Thomas L. DesMarais, Zhaohui Tong, Yixin Yao, and Max Costa, "Oxidative Stress Alters Global Histone Modification and DNA Methylation," *Free Radical Biology and Medicine* 82 (2015): 22-28.

194   Xin Yi, et al., "Histone Methylation and Oxidative Stress in Cardiovascular Diseases," *Oxidative Medicine and Cellular Longevity* (2022); Yi, "Histone Methylation and Oxidative Stress."

195   Thomas Kietzmann, et al., "The Epigenetic Landscape Related to Reactive Oxygen Species Formation in the Cardiovascular System," *British Journal of Pharmacology* 174, no. 12 (2017): 1533-1554; Kurek, Katarzyna, Beata Plitta-Michalak, and Ewelina Ratajczak, "Reactive Oxygen Species as Potential Drivers of the Seed Aging Process," *Plants* 8, no. 6 (2019): 174.

196   Cyrus Martin and Yi Zhang, "Mechanisms of Epigenetic Inheritance," *Current Opinion in Cell Biology* 19, no. 3 (2007): 266-272; Millissia Ben Maamar, Ingrid Sadler-Riggleman, Daniel Beck, and Michael K. Skinner, "Epigenetic Transgenerational Inheritance of Altered Sperm Histone Retention Sites," *Scientific Reports* 8, no. 1 (2018): 5308; Bing Zhu and Danny Reinberg, "Epigenetic Inheritance: Uncontested?" *Cell Research* 21, no. 3 (2011): 435-441.

197   Thelma M. Escobar, et al., "Inheritance of Repressed Chromatin Domains during S Phase Requires the Histone Chaperone NPM1," *Science Advances* 8, no. 17 (2022): Eabm3945.

198   Jason H. Brickner, "Inheritance of Epigenetic Transcriptional Memory through Read–Write Replication of a Histone Modification," *Annals of the New York Academy of Sciences* (2023); Pauline N. C. B. Audergon, et al., "Restricted Epigenetic Inheritance of H3K9 Methylation," *Science* 348, no. 6230 (2015): 132–135; Jason H. Brickner, "Inheritance of Epigenetic Transcriptional Memory through Read–Write Replication of a Histone Modification," *Annals of the New York Academy of Sciences* (2023).

199   Christopher I. Cazzonelli, Tony Millar, E. Jean Finnegan, and Barry J. Pogson, "Promoting Gene Expression in Plants by Permissive Histone Lysine Methylation," *Plant Signaling & Behavior* 4, no. 6 (2009): 484–488; Michael Chas Sumner and Jason Brickner, "The Nuclear Pore Complex as a Transcription Regulator," *Cold Spring Harbor Perspectives in Biology* 14, no. 1 (2022): A039438; André Hoelz, Erik W. Debler, and Günter Blobel, "The Structure of the Nuclear Pore Complex," *Annual Review of Biochemistry* 80 (2011): 613–643; Bethany Sump and Jason Brickner, "Establishment and Inheritance of Epigenetic Transcriptional Memory," *Frontiers in Molecular Biosciences* 9 (2022): 977653; Michael Chas Sumner and Jason Brickner, "The Nuclear Pore Complex as a Transcription Regulator," *Cold Spring Harbor Perspectives in Biology* 14, no. 1 (2022): A039438.

200   Gilbert S. Omenn, "Reflections on the HUPO Human Proteome Project, the Flagship Project of the Human Proteome Organization, at 10 Years," *Molecular & Cellular Proteomics* 20 (2021); James R. Iben and Richard J. Maraia, "tRNA Gene Copy Number Variation in Humans," *Gene* 536, no. 2 (2014): 376–384.

201   Ran Elkon and Reuven Agami, "Characterization of Noncoding Regulatory DNA in the Human Genome," *Nature Biotechnology* 35, no. 8 (2017): 732–746; Kevin V. Morris and John S. Mattick, "The Rise of Regulatory RNA," *Nature Reviews Genetics* 15, no. 6 (2014): 423–437; Julia Höck and Gunter Meister, "The Argonaute Protein Family," *Genome Biology* 9 (2008): 1–8; Hotaka Kobayashi and Yukihide Tomari, "RISC Assembly: Coordination between Small RNAs and Argonaute Proteins," *Biochimica Et Biophysica Acta (BBA)-Gene Regulatory Mechanisms* 1859, no. 1 (2016): 71–81; Kotaro Nakanishi, "Anatomy of RISC: How Do Small RNAs and Chaperones Activate Argonaute Proteins?" *Wiley Interdisciplinary Reviews: RNA* 7, no. 5 (2016): 637–660.

202   Y. Lee, K-H Jinju Han, Jin H. Yeo, and V. N. Kim, "Drosha in Primary MicroRNA Processing," *Cold Spring Harbor Symposia on Quantitative Biology* 71 (2006): 51–57; Ashley M. Mohr and Justin L. Mott, "Overview of MicroRNA Biology," *Seminars in Liver Disease* 35, no. 1 (2015): 3–11.

203   Yoontae Lee, et al., "The Nuclear RNase III Drosha Initiates MicroRNA Processing," *Nature* 425, no. 6956 (2003): 415–419; Ahmet M. Denli, et al., "Processing of Primary MicroRNAs by the Microprocessor Complex," *Nature* 432, no. 7014 (2004): 231–235.

204   Rui Yi, Yi Qin, Ian G. Macara, and Bryan R. Cullen, "Exportin-5 Mediates the Nuclear Export of Pre-MicroRNAs and Short Hairpin RNAs," *Genes & Development* 17, no. 24 (2003): 3011–3016; Lukasz Jaskiewicz and Witold Filipowicz, "Role of Dicer in Posttranscriptional RNA Silencing," *RNA Interference* (2008): 77–97.

205   Marc R. Fabian and Nahum Sonenberg, "The Mechanics of miRNA-Mediated Gene Silencing: A Look under the Hood of miRISC," *Nature Structural & Molecular Biology* 19, no. 6 (2012): 586–593; Hotaka Kobayashi and Yukihide Tomari, "RISC Assembly: Coordination Between Small RNAs and Argonaute Proteins," *Biochimica Et Biophysica Acta (BBA)-Gene Regulatory Mechanisms* 1859, no. 1 (2016): 71–81; Ashley J. Pratt and Ian J. Macrae, "The RNA-Induced Silencing Complex: A Versatile Gene-Silencing Machine," *Journal of Biological Chemistry* 284, no. 27 (2009): 17897–17901.

206   Richard I.Gregory, Thimmaiah P. Chendrimada, Neil Cooch, and Ramin Shiekhattar, "Human RISC Couples MicroRNA Biogenesis and Posttranscriptional Gene Silencing," *Cell* 123, no. 4 (2005): 631–640.

207   Frank J. Slack, "Regulatory RNAs and the Demise of 'Junk' DNA," (2006): 1–2; Samuel Corless, Saskia Höcker, and Sylvia Erhardt, "Centromeric RNA and Its Function at and Beyond Centromeric Chromatin," *Journal of Molecular Biology* 432, no. 15 (2020): 4257–4269; Daniel Stoyko, Pavol Genzor, and Astrid D. Haase, "Hierarchical Length and Sequence Preferences Establish a Single Major piRNA 3'-End," *Iscience* 25, no. 6 (2022); Celina Juliano, Jianquan Wang, and Haifan Lin, "Uniting Germline and Stem Cells: The Function of Piwi Proteins and the PiRNA Pathway in Diverse Organisms," *Annual Review of Genetics* 45 (2011): 447–469.

208   Yu H. Sun, et al., "Coupled Protein Synthesis and Ribosome-Guided PiRNA Processing on mRNAs," *Nature Communications* 12, no. 1 (2021):

5970; Dansen Wu, et al., "Effects of Novel ncRNA Molecules, p15-piRNAs, on the Methylation of DNA and Histone H3 of the CDKN2B Promoter Region in U937 Cells," *Journal of Cellular Biochemistry* 116, no. 12 (2015): 2744–2754; Jaspreet S. Khurana and William Theurkauf, "piRNAs, Transposon Silencing, and Drosophila Germline Development," *Journal of Cell Biology* 191, no. 5 (2010): 905–913.

209 Jiajia Wang, et al., "Pirbase: A Comprehensive Database of piRNA Sequences," *Nucleic Acids Research* 47, no. D1 (2019): D175–D180.

210 Nathaniel C. Comfort, "From Controlling Elements to Transposons: Barbara McClintock and the Nobel Prize," *TRENDS In Genetics* 17, no. 8 (2001): 475–478; Corentin Claeys Bouuaert and Ronald M. Chalmers, "Gene Therapy Vectors: The Prospects and Potentials of the Cut-and-Paste Transposons," *Genetica* 138 (2010): 473–484; Lukas Schrader and Jürgen Schmitz, "The Impact of Transposable Elements in Adaptive Evolution," *Molecular Ecology* 28, no. 6 (2019): 1537–1549; Cédric Feschotte and Ellen J. Pritham, "DNA Transposons and the Evolution of Eukaryotic Genomes," *Annual Review of Genetics* 41 (2007): 331–368.

211 Ozge Cemiloglu Ulker, et al., "Short Overview on the Relevance pf MicroRNA–Reactive Oxygen Species (ROS) Interactions and Lipid Peroxidation for Modulation of Oxidative Stress-Mediated Signalling Pathways in Cancer Treatment," *Journal of Pharmacy and Pharmacology* 74, no. 4 (2022): 503–515; Jun He and Bing-Hua Jiang, "Interplay Between Reactive Oxygen Species and MicroRNAs in Cancer," *Current Pharmacology Reports* 2, no. 2 (2016): 82–90; Valeria Villarreal-García, et al., "A Vicious Circle in Breast Cancer: The Interplay Between Inflammation, Reactive Oxygen Species, and MicroRNAs," *Frontiers in Oncology* 12 (2022): 980694; Yao-Yu Gong, Jiang-Yun Luo, Li Wang, and Yu Huang, "MicroRNAs Regulating Reactive Oxygen Species in Cardiovascular Diseases," *Antioxidants & Redox Signaling* 29, no. 11 (2018): 1092–1107.

212 Jaideep Banerjee, Savita Khanna, and Akash Bhattacharya, "MicroRNA Regulation of Oxidative Stress," *Oxidative Medicine and Cellular Longevity* (2017).

213 Julia Konovalova, et al., "Interplay Between MicroRNAs and Oxidative Stress in Neurodegenerative Diseases," *International Journal of Molecular Sciences* 20, no. 23 (2019): 6055.

214   Irene Pedersen and Michael David, "MicroRNAs in the Immune Response," *Cytokine* 43, no. 3 (2008): 391–394; Enikö Sonkoly and Andor Pivarcsi, "MicroRNAs in Inflammation," *International Reviews of Immunology* 28, no. 6 (2009): 535–561; Mark M. Perry, et al., "Rapid Changes in MicroRNA-146a Expression Negatively Regulate The IL-1β-Induced Inflammatory Response in Human Lung Alveolar Epithelial Cells," *The Journal of Immunology* 180, no. 8 (2008): 5689–5698; Huimin Kong, et al., "The Effect of miR-132, miR-146a, and miR-155 on MRP8/TLR4 Astrocyte-Related Inflammation," *Journal of Molecular Neuroscience* 57 (2015): 28–37; Maurizio Ceppi, et al., "MicroRNA-155 Modulates the Interleukin-1 Signaling Pathway in Activated Human Monocyte-Derived Dendritic Cells," *Proceedings of the National Academy of Sciences* 106, no. 8 (2009): 2735–2740; Shuo Li, Yan Yue, Wei Xu, and Sidong Xiong, "MicroRNA-146a Represses Mycobacteria-Induced Inflammatory Response and Facilitates Bacterial Replication via Targeting IRAK-1 And TRAF-6," *PloS One* 8, no. 12 (2013): E81438; Natheer H. Al-Rawi, et al., "Salivary MicroRNA 155, 146a/B and 203: A Pilot Study for Potentially Non-Invasive Diagnostic Biomarkers of Periodontitis and Diabetes Mellitus," *PloS One* 15, no. 8 (2020): E0237004.

215   Iftach Shaked, et al., "MicroRNA-132 Potentiates Cholinergic Anti-Inflammatory Signaling by Targeting Acetylcholinesterase," *Immunity* 31, no. 6 (2009): 965–973.

216   Haomin Yan, et al., "miRNA-132/212 Regulates Tight Junction Stabilization in Blood-Brain Barrier after Stroke," *Cell Death Discovery* 7, no. 1 (2021): 380; Zheng Gang Zhang, Benjamin Buller, and Michael Chopp, "Exosomes–Beyond Stem Cells for Restorative Therapy in Stroke and Neurological Injury," *Nature Reviews Neurology* 15, no. 4 (2019): 193–203.

217   Ying Jiang, et al., "miR-210 Mediates Vagus Nerve Stimulation-Induced Antioxidant Stress and Anti-Apoptosis Reactions Following Cerebral Ischemia/Reperfusion Injury in Rats," *Journal of Neurochemistry* 134, no. 1 (2015): 173–181.

218   Yang Sun, et al., "MicroRNA-124 Mediates the Cholinergic Anti-Inflammatory Action through Inhibiting the Production of Pro-Inflammatory Cytokines," *Cell Research* 23, no. 11 (2013): 1270–1283; Luis Ulloa, "The Cholinergic Anti-Inflammatory Pathway Meets MicroRNA," *Cell Research* 23, no. 11 (2013): 1249–1250; Bettina Nadorp and Hermona Soreq, "Predicted Overlapping MicroRNA Regulators of Acetylcholine

Packaging and Degradation in Neuroinflammation-Related Disorders," *Frontiers in Molecular Neuroscience* 7 (2014): 9.

219 Laura Musazzi, et al., "Stress, MicroRNAs, and Stress-Related Psychiatric Disorders: An Overview," *Molecular Psychiatry* (2023): 1–18; Shan Huang, et al., "Increased miR-124-3p In Microglial Exosomes Following Traumatic Brain Injury Inhibits Neuronal Inflammation and Contributes to Neurite Outgrowth via Their Transfer into Neurons," *The FASEB Journal* 32, no. 1 (2018): 512–528; Yongxiang Yang, et al., "miR-124 Enriched Exosomes Promoted the M2 Polarization of Microglia and Enhanced Hippocampus Neurogenesis after Traumatic Brain Injury by Inhibiting TLR4 Pathway," *Neurochemical Research* 44 (2019): 811–828.

220 Uriya Bekenstein, et al., "Dynamic Changes in Murine Forebrain mir-211 Expression Associate with Cholinergic Imbalances and Epileptiform Activity," *Proceedings of the National Academy of Sciences* 114, no. 25 (2017): E4996–E5005; Katherine A. Halawa, et al., "Molecular, Physiological and Behavioral Characterization of the Heterozygous Df [H15q13]/+ Mouse Model Associated with the Human 15q13. 3 Microdeletion Syndrome," *Brain Research* 1746 (2020): 147024; Uriya Bekenstein, et al., "Dynamic Changes in Murine Forebrain miR-211 Expression Associate with Cholinergic Imbalances and Epileptiform Activity," *Proceedings of the National Academy of Sciences* 114, no. 25 (2017): E4996–E5005.

221 Teresa H. Sanders, et al., "Cognition-Enhancing Vagus Nerve Stimulation Alters the Epigenetic Landscape," *Journal of Neuroscience* 39, no. 18 (2019): 3454–3469.

222 Carlos López-Otín, et al., "The Hallmarks of Aging," *Cell* 153, no. 6 (2013): 1194–1217.

223 Al Aboud, Nora M., Connor Tupper, and Ishwarlal Jialal, "Genetics, Epigenetic Mechanism," in *Statpearls*, St. Petersburg, FL: Statpearls Publishing, 2022; Irene Hernando-Herraez, Raquel Garcia-Perez, Andrew J. Sharp, and Tomas Marques-Bonet, "DNA Methylation: Insights into Human Evolution," *Plos Genetics* 11, no. 12 (2015): E1005661; Pamela E. Bennett-Baker, Jodi Wilkowski, and David T. Burke, "Age-Associated Activation of Epigenetically Repressed Genes in the Mouse," *Genetics* 165, no. 4 (2003): 2055–2062; Stella Marie Reamon-Buettner, Vanessa Mutschler, and Juergen Borlak, "The Next Innovation Cycle in Toxicogenomics: Environmental Epigenetics," *Mutation Research/*

Reviews in Mutation Research 659, no. 12 (2008): 158-165; Randall S. Gieni, Ismail H. Ismail, Stuart Campbell, and Michael J. Hendzel, "Polycomb Group Proteins in the DNA Damage Response: A Link Between Radiation Resistance and 'Stemness,'" *Cell Cycle* 10, no. 6 (2011): 883-894; Shufei Song and F. Brad Johnson, "Epigenetic Mechanisms Impacting Aging: A Focus on Histone Levels and Telomeres," *Genes* 9, no. 4 (2018): 201; Navneet K. Matharu and Rakesh K. Mishra, "Tone Up Your Chromatin and Stay Young," *Journal of Biosciences* 36 (2011): 5-11.

224   Gawain McColl, et al., "Pharmacogenetic Analysis of Lithium-Induced Delayed Aging in Caenorhabditis Elegans," *Journal of Biological Chemistry* 283, no. 1 (2008): 350-357.

225   Travis J. Maures, Eric L. Greer, Anna G. Hauswirth, and Anne Brunet, "The H3K27 Demethylase UTX-1 Regulates C. Elegans Lifespan in a Germline-Independent, Insulin-Dependent Manner," *Aging Cell* 10, no. 6 (2011): 980-990.

226   Kathrine B. Dall and Nils J. Færgeman, "Metabolic Regulation of Lifespan from A. C. Elegans Perspective," *Genes & Nutrition* 14, no. 1 (2019): 1-12; Teresa Lee, et al., "Repressive H3K9me2 Protects Lifespan Against the Transgenerational Burden of COMPASS Activity in C. Elegans," *Elife* 8 (2019): E48498.

227   Dae-Sung Hwangbo, Hye-Yeon Lee, Leen Suleiman Abozaid, and Kyung-Jin Min, "Mechanisms of Lifespan Regulation by Calorie Restriction and Intermittent Fasting in Model Organisms," *Nutrients* 12, no. 4 (2020): 1194; Diego Hernández-Saavedra, Laura Moody, Guanying Bianca Xu, Hong Chen, and Yuan-Xiang Pan, "Epigenetic Regulation of Metabolism and Inflammation by Calorie Restriction," *Advances in Nutrition* 10, no. 3 (2019): 520-536; Ki Wung Chung and Hae Young Chung, "The Effects of Calorie Restriction on Autophagy: Role on Aging Intervention," *Nutrients* 11, no. 12 (2019): 2923.

228   Weiya Cao, Jinhong Li, Kepeng Yang, and Dongli Cao, "An Overview of Autophagy: Mechanism, Regulation, and Research Progress," *Bulletin Du Cancer* 108, no. 3 (2021): 304-322; Nerea Deleyto-Seldas and Alejo Efeyan, "The mTOR-Autophagy Axis and the Control of Metabolism," *Frontiers in Cell and Developmental Biology* 9 (2021): 655731.

229   Kathrin Schmeisser and J. Alex Parker, "Pleiotropic Effects of mTOR and Autophagy during Development and Aging," *Frontiers in Cell and Developmental Biology* 7 (2019): 192; Ying Wang and Hongbing Zhang,

"Regulation of Autophagy by mTOR Signaling Pathway," *Autophagy: Biology and Diseases: Basic Science* (2019): 67–83.

230 Diego Molina-Serrano, Dimitris Kyriakou, and Antonis Kirmizis, "Histone Modifications as an Intersection Between Diet and Longevity," *Frontiers in Genetics* 10 (2019): 192.

231 Patricia González-Rodríguez, Jens Füllgrabe, and Bertrand Joseph, "The Hunger Strikes Back: An Epigenetic Memory for Autophagy," *Cell Death & Differentiation* (2023): 1–12.

232 Akshay Bareja, David E. Lee, and James P. White, "Maximizing Longevity and Healthspan: Multiple Approaches All Converging on Autophagy," *Frontiers in Cell and Developmental Biology* 7 (2019): 183.

233 Sing-Hua Tsou, "Dietary Restriction and mTOR and IIS Inhibition: The Potential to Antiaging Drug Approach," *Anti-Aging Drug Discovery on the Basis of Hallmarks of Aging* (2022): 173–190.

234 Ji Yong Kim, David Mondaca-Ruff, Sandeep Singh, and Yu Wang, "SIRT1 and Autophagy: Implications in Endocrine Disorders," *Frontiers in Endocrinology* 13 (2022): 930919; Yoomi Chun and Joungmok Kim, "Ampk-mTOR Signaling and Cellular Adaptations in Hypoxia," *International Journal of Molecular Sciences* 22, no. 18 (2021): 9765.

235 Chiara Vidoni, et al., "Calorie Restriction for Cancer Prevention and Therapy: Mechanisms, Expectations, and Efficacy," *Journal of Cancer Prevention* 26, no. 4 (2021): 224.

236 Diego Hernández-Saavedra, et al., "Epigenetic Regulation of Metabolism and Inflammation by Calorie Restriction," *Advances in Nutrition* 10, no. 3 (2019): 520–536.

237 Yunus Akkoc, and Devrim Gozuacik, "MicroRNAs as Major Regulators of the Autophagy Pathway," *Biochimica Et Biophysica Acta (BBA)-Molecular Cell Research* 1867, no. 5 (2020): 118662.

238 Chan Shan et al., "The Emerging Roles of Autophagy-Related MicroRNAs in Cancer," *International Journal of Biological Sciences* 17, no. 1 (2021): 134; Sounak Ghosh Roy, "Regulation of Autophagy by miRNAs in Human Diseases," *The Nucleus* 64, no. 3 (2021): 317–329.

239 Bizhou Bie, et al., "Vagus Nerve Stimulation Affects Inflammatory Response and Anti-Apoptosis Reactions via Regulating miR-210 in Epilepsy Rat Model," *Neuroreport* 32, no. 9 (2021): 783–791; Andrew Fesler, et al., "Autophagy Regulated by miRNAs in Colorectal Cancer Progression and Resistance," *Cancer Translational Medicine* 3, no. 3 (2017): 96; T-X. Xu,

S-Z. Zhao, M. Dong, and X-R. Yu, "Hypoxia Responsive miR-210 Promotes Cell Survival and Autophagy of Endometriotic Cells in Hypoxia," *European Review for Medical & Pharmacological Sciences* 20, no. 3 (2016); Cheng Wang, et al., "miR-210 Facilitates ECM Degradation by Suppressing Autophagy via Silencing of ATG7 in Human Degenerated NP Cells," *Biomedicine & Pharmacotherapy* 93 (2017): 470–479.

240 Alexander Graham Bell, *The Duration of Life and Conditions Associated with Longevity: A Study of the Hyde Genealogy*, San Francisco: Genealogical Record Office, 1918; Albert I. Lansing, "A Transmissible, Cumulative, and Reversible Factor in Aging," *Journal of Gerontology* 2, no. 3 (1947): 228–239; Charles E. King, "A Re-Examination of the Lansing Effect," *Biology of Rotifers* (1983): 135–139.

241 Elmar W. Tobi, et al., "DNA Methylation Signatures Link Prenatal Famine Exposure to Growth and Metabolism," *Nature Communications* 5, no. 1 (2014): 5592; Patricia González-Rodríguez, Jens Füllgrabe, and Bertrand Joseph, "The Hunger Strikes Back: An Epigenetic Memory for Autophagy," *Cell Death & Differentiation* (2023): 1–12; Lars Olov Bygren, Gunnar Kaati, and Sören Edvinsson, "Longevity Determined by Paternal Ancestors' Nutrition during Their Slow Growth Period," *Acta Biotheoretica* 49 (2001): 53–59.

242 Li-Fang Hu, "Epigenetic Regulation of Autophagy," *Autophagy: Biology and Diseases: Basic Science* (2019): 221–236.

243 Huan Wang, *Autophagy: Activation, Function and Regulation by a Protein Restricted Diet during Pregnancy and Lactation*, Chicago: University of Illinois at Urbana-Champaign, 2015; Lei Qiu, Xueqin Liu, and Junhong Han, "Maternally Inherited H4K16 Acetylation Primes Zygotic Gene Activation in Drosophila," *Science China Life Sciences* 63 (2020): 1950–1952; Agnieszka Gadecka and Anna Bielak-Zmijewska, "Slowing Down Ageing: The Role of Nutrients and Microbiota in Modulation of the Epigenome," *Nutrients* 11, no. 6 (2019): 1251.

244 Wilfred Roo, "Micro-RNAs as Regulators of Senescence and Aging," Faculty of Science and Engineering, 2012.

245 Alexandre Champroux, et al., "Preimplantation Embryos Amplify Sperm-Derived miRNA Levels to Mediate Transgenerational Epigenetic Inheritance," *bioRxiv* (2023): 2023-04.

246   Gursoy-Ozdemir, et al.,"Cortical Spreading Depression Activates and Upregulates MMP-9," *The Journal of Clinical Investigation,* 113, no. 10 (2004): 1447–1455.

247   Brebner, et al.,"Synergistic Effects of Interleukin-1β, Interleukin-6, and Tumor Necrosis Factor-α" *Neuropsychopharmacology* 22, no. 6 (2000): 566–580.; Zhu, et al., "The Proinflammatory Cytokines Interleukin-1beta and Tumor Necrosis Factor-Alpha Activate Serotonin Transporters," *Neuropsychopharmacology* 31, no. 10 (2006): 2121–2131.

248   Ricci, et al., "Astrocyte–Neuron Interactions in Neurological Disorders," *The Journal of Biological Physics* 35 (2009): 317–336; Hansson, et al., "Glial Neuronal Signaling in the Central Nervous System," *FASEB Journal* 17, no. 3 (2003): 341–348; Zou, et al., "TNFα Potentiates Glutamate Neurotoxicity by Inhibiting Glutamate Uptake in Organotypic Brain Slice Cultures," *Brain Research* 1034, no. 1–2 (2005): 11–24; Pickering, et al., "Actions of TNF-α on Glutamatergic Synaptic Transmission in the Central Nervous System," *Experimental Physiology* 90, no. 5 (2005): 663–670.

ACKNOWLEDGMENTS

To individually thank everyone who has helped me acquire the knowledge I am sharing in this book would be impossible, and yet not to attempt to do so would be a sin. Therefore, forgive me, in advance, for any omissions.

First, I must thank my loving wife, Leigh Ann, for her unwavering support of my pursuit of the truth. Her will to see that I share it with the world is the force that made this work reality. I love you and our children, Samantha, Thomas, Charlotte, and Nicolas, more than anything. Thank you for being my partner in life. We will make the world a happier, healthier, and smarter place for all.

Next, I am so happy to acknowledge and thank my friend and intellectual confidant, Bruce Simon, without whom I would have stumbled aimlessly around in the dark for decades. The years spent sparring with you in our offices shaped me in so many positive ways, and along the way lit a path to a healthier world for all. If we were trapped in the Library of Babel for near eternity, it would not be enough time to test the potential of your intellect, plumb the depths of your curiosity, or exhaust your generosity of spirit.

This book would literally not exist were if not for Dr. Navaz Habib, my cohost on *The Health Upgrade Podcast*. What was originally supposed to be a twenty-minute call has turned into a partnership that has opened my eyes to many things, and given me the faith to believe the conclusions my mind had been drawing for years. You are a good man, and I am happy to have partnered with you to make this a better world.

I would be remiss were I not to acknowledge and thank all those who have sparred with me, and even challenged my beliefs and conclusions over the past twenty years. Whether we agreed or disagreed, you made me question what I thought was true and forced me to come to stronger conclusions, no matter what sacred calves needed to be sacrificed along the way. Some names for the record books include Dr. Kevin Tracey, Dr. Peter Goadsby, Dr. Zam Cader, Dr. Cenk Ayata, Dr. David Yoder, Dr. Marie-Eve Tremblay, Dr. Michael Oshinsky, Dr. Josef Gorek, Dr. Adam Farmer, Dr. Owen Epstein, Dr. Nicholas Silver, and Dr. Paul Durham.

Finally, to my business partners, Dr. Peter Staats, Dr. Thomas Errico, and Dr. Charles Theofilos: Thank you for affording me the opportunity to learn while doing. In the words of Winston Churchill, "Now this is not the end. It is not even the beginning of the end. But it is, perhaps, the end of the beginning."

ABOUT THE AUTHOR

JP Errico is a highly accomplished individual with a diverse range of expertise as an executive, entrepreneur, and inventor. He has founded and served in various capacities, ranging from CEO and board member to chief science officer and key consultant, for a number of public and private healthcare companies. Most recently, JP has served as a board member of ElectroCore, a NASDAQ-listed company (ECOR) that he founded in 2005. ElectroCore specializes in neuromodulation technologies, including a noninvasive vagus nerve stimulator that JP coinvented in 2010.

JP has been credited as an inventor on over 250 issued US patents, and has founded and successfully sold or taken public numerous medical device and pharmaceutical companies, in partnership with Dr. Thomas J. Errico and others. These companies include Fastenetix, K2 Medical Systems, AD4-Pharma, E2, and SpineCor. He has served on the boards of Oculogica and Morphogenesis and is currently advising Ondine Biomedical. He earned an undergraduate degree in aeronautical engineering from the Massachusetts Institute of Technology and worked at the Air Force National Laboratory's Lincoln Laboratories. Additionally, he holds graduate degrees in both law and mechanical/materials engineering from Duke University.

JP has contributed several book chapters to medical textbooks, including *Neuromodulation* 2nd ed., and is the cohost of *The Health Upgrade Podcast* with Dr. Navaz Habib, author of *Activate Your Vagus Nerve* and *Upgrade Your Vagus Nerve*. He is a frequent expert guest on *Healthcare Summits*, produced by DrTalks, covering topics ranging from mitochondrial health and inflammation to neurodegenerative disorders and metabolic health. In addition, he has developed a groundbreaking program, Overcoming Chronic Threat Response Mode, which is available through a variety of channels, including his website, JPErrico.com. His blog posts and other writings can also be found there.